I'M FULL

Remindful Eating Tips to Feel Great
and Make Peace with your Plate

Theresa Yosuico Stahl,
RDN, LDN, FAND

Theresa Stahl

Wishing you a full life,
Theresa Stahl

I'm Full: Remindful Eating Tips to Feel Great and Make Peace with your Plate

ISBN: 978-1-7378688-7-3

Published in the United States of America by:

Theresa Stahl

To order a copy of this book, please visit:

https://www.remindfuleating.com/

Disclaimer: Information contained in this book is for general education. No information, written or implied, is intended to be considered medical advice for any individual. Please consult your own medical professionals regarding any individual medical and nutrition advice.

Trademark notice: This book uses various trademarked names, within its text. In the interest of the reader, we are using the trademarked names in an editorial style. In the interest of the trademark holders, we cite their ownership of the trademarks, with no intention of infringement.

Time sensitive materials: At the time of publication, all names, addresses, telephone numbers, email and web addresses were verified as accurate.

To my beloved children, Sarah and Benjamin:

May you always grow, be inspired, and inspire others.

***

CONTENTS

INTRODUCTION

For the Love of Food

Food, glorious food!
Eat right through the menu.
Just loosen your belt
Two inches and then you
Work up a new appetite.
In this interlude --
The food,
Once again, food,
Fabulous food,
Glorious food.

Lionel Bart from the play Oliver!

As early as I can remember, I have loved food. I feel excited at the thought of my next meal. My best and first food memories began in my grandmother's kitchen. Her long, wooden spoon seemed magical in my hands. I would lift the lid on the enormous pot of simmering tomato sauce, place the spoon into the pot, and stir. Steam would rise like a cloud of smoke and the rich aroma filled my senses. The meatballs were like buried treasure under the sea of sauce.

My grandparents, Antonia and Sabatino, traveled to America from San Lorenzo Nuovo, Italy. They came on their honeymoon and never left. They had seven children, raised their own chickens, and grew an extensive vegetable garden. Right beside the garden was a large grape arbor with a bench swing built under it. Countless hours were spent swinging with my sister and cousins -- singing, talking, and laughing. The sweet scent of grapes encircled us as we made memories filled with food and fun.

On Sundays, we attended Mass, then stopped by the local bookstore to browse. My mom bought me the latest issue of a magazine or comic book, along with a few pieces of penny candy. Afterwards, it was off to my grandparents for dinner. I always arrived with a huge appetite feeling like I was starving. My mom joked with others that my stomach was a "bottomless pit." I must admit that I did have an extra-large appetite for such a tiny, little girl. I loved food! And there always seemed to be room for more.

I believe my metabolism and boundless energy helped me maintain a healthy weight during my childhood. I was always active – riding bikes, running, dancing, gymnastics, swimming, and tennis. We were the generation of kids who played outside all day and all night without any fear of harm. My neighborhood was my playground and I loved playing with my neighborhood friends. I lived beside a middle school, so I had a large parking lot for bike riding, fields for running, and the side of the school's huge brick wall for hitting tennis balls.

My overeating habits caught up with me in my first year of college in the form of the "freshman 15." As I ate a steady diet of the two items my school cafeteria did well – hot homemade rolls and hand-dipped ice cream – the freshman 15 became the freshman 20. Frightened by the prospect of that 20 turning into 30 or more, I became interested in healthy eating. Obesity runs in my family, as does high cholesterol, high blood pressure, heart disease, and diabetes. If I didn't do something now, I feared, nature would take its genetic course.

My father was a doctor, and my mother was a nurse, but I didn't like the sight of blood, so neither career path appealed to me. Nutrition combined the medical world I grew up in with my love of food. I loved studying the science of nutrition and the role food played in health, so I became a registered dietitian nutritionist (RDN). I guess you could say I followed in the footsteps of Hippocrates, the father of medicine, who said, "Let food be thy medicine and let medicine be thy food."

Over the course of 40 years, I have been fortunate to help thousands of clients and students find their way to a healthier lifestyle. Family, friends, and strangers alike pick my brain for nutrition tips. So, I decided to compile the tips that have worked best for me and those I've served. My goal is to inspire, motivate, and educate in an easy-to-read book. Read the tips in sequence or skip around. Each tip concludes with a section called Dig Deeper. This section contains items for self-reflection and action steps to move you forward. It also contains resources used in writing the tip and recommended reading for more information on the tip topic. I hope you enjoy this collection of what I have learned so far.

PART ONE: HUNGER, FULLNESS, AND MINDFUL EATING

* * *

TIP 1 - THE POWER OF SAYING "I'M FULL."

"I can't get no satisfaction, but I try, yes I try."

Mick Jagger and Keith Richards, The Rolling Stones

Originally written in 1965 as a statement against commercialism and the status-quo, this song's pulsating chorus captures the feeling experienced by many every day. It's no wonder that it has a prominent place as number 2 on Rolling Stone magazine's list of the 500 Greatest Songs of All Time.

What is satisfaction and why is it so elusive? Is anyone ever truly satisfied? Is there even such a thing as achieving satisfaction? And if so, what does it look like, how does it feel, and how does it impact one's life?

The Merriam-Webster dictionary defines satisfaction as the fulfillment of a need or want; a source or means of enjoyment. Contentment and gratification are used to describe the state of being satisfied.

We find strong links among satisfaction, contentment, gratification, and fulfillment. This applies to all areas of our lives, including our eating habits and weight control. This is what has led me to call this book **"I'm Full."**

These simple words hold a lot of power. Saying them empowers you. There's commitment and resolution in these words. When you say them, you are making not just an observation, but also a decision that allows you to execute self-control; not just about eating, but about life as well.

Saying "I'm full" helps me solidify my own boundaries with food. Growing up, I routinely ate until I was stuffed. I thought that it was how one was supposed to feel at the end of a meal, just like many of my clients. Children are the most honest. When asked, "How do you know when to stop eating?" They often respond, "When my tummy hurts."

Can you imagine the powerful effect of teaching ourselves, our children, our grandchildren, and others to say proudly:

"I'm full."
"I'm satisfied."
"I'm content."
"Yes, I am. Full."

Dig Deeper

Reflection and action:

1. Do you pay attention to how you feel when you're eating?

2. This week, practice saying, "I'm full," "I'm satisfied," and "I'm content," and put your fork down. Focus on how you feel at different points in your meal.

TIP 2 - USE A PERIOD INSTEAD OF A BUT ...

"Do it today, because sometimes later becomes never."

Karen Salmansohn, self-help author

Too often the words "I'm full" are followed up with a great big BUT. "I'm full, BUT I'm going to eat more anyway," or "I'm full, but I can't let food go to waste because there are starving children in the world." Was this logic used by your parents? Do you feel guilty leaving food on your plate? Do you think you are wasting food, so you clean your plate, just like you were taught?

Here are some reasons I hear for eating beyond the point of satisfaction or fullness:

- "I'm full, but it tastes so good, I just can't stop eating." Some foods taste so good that it's easy to go overboard. How about those donuts that just melt in your mouth? They go down so easily, but with over 200 calories each, it's easy to overdo it.

- "I'm full, but I don't know when I will eat again, so I better eat all I can now." Did you or your parents grow up during the Great Depression? Did you or your parents experience food insecurity, not having enough food for the whole family? If there wasn't or isn't enough food to go around, it's "everyone for themselves" when it comes to getting enough to eat.

- "I'm full, but I'm starting a diet tomorrow, so I better eat all I want now." This is called "last supper" thinking. Have you ever justified overeating since this is the last time you will be enjoying a normal meal for a long time because you're starting a diet tomorrow? Maybe you are like many others who routinely start and stop diets. If so, then the number of "last suppers" add up over the years, as do the pounds from yo-yo dieting. This unfortunate diet cycle of losing while on a diet and gaining when off the diet, often results in a higher weight than before the cycle began. This is documented in many studies. This weight cycling continues until you decide to give up dieting, in exchange for a lifetime of healthier, mindful eating habits.

- "I'm full, but I'm drowning my sorrows, anger, or stress." Have you ever seen the recipe for "break-up" brownies? It reads, "Prepare brownies according to box directions and eat the whole pan while crying." While this was meant to be humorous, too many people use food as comfort and despite the momentary rise in brain chemicals, such as serotonin, associated with feeling better, the unwanted weight gain brings more stress, shame, and anger in the long run.

- "I'm full, but there's always room for dessert." According to research, no matter how full a person may be, one can make room for dessert. This is due to what is called the "mindless margin," which is the margin in which we can decide to overeat or undereat by about 20%, without noticing the differences.

Today, let's leave the "buts" behind and learn to consistently say with conviction, "I'm full." That's it. Just simply, "I'm full." Meal after meal. You will see an amazing transformation in your thinking and behavior. These two words really can help you put an end to overeating, help you enjoy your favorite foods, and gain control of your weight forever. The upcoming tips will help you learn how.

Dig Deeper

Reflection and action:

1. What are the "buts" that are holding you back from feeling full? Write them on a piece of paper and resolve to leave those "buts" behind. After you write these down, crumple up the paper and toss it into the trash to symbolize the end of this behavior.

2. This week, listen carefully to yourself – do you hear any "buts" to "I'm full?" If you do, say "I'm full, period. No buts."

Resources and reading:

1. Wansink, B. (2011). *Mindless eating: Why we eat more than we think.* Hay House.

TIP 3 - THINK "GLASS HALF-FULL"

*"Optimism is the faith that leads to achievement.
Nothing can be done without hope and confidence."*

Helen Keller, author, disability rights activist

Situations experienced in life are seen differently by different people.

Two men looked out from prison bars. One saw mud and the other stars. Two sons grew up with an alcoholic father. One became an alcoholic and blamed it on his dad. The other never drank alcohol because he didn't want to be like his dad.

How one responds to situations influences outcomes. How about you? Do you see the glass as half full or half empty?

Your answer to this simple question has far reaching implications. Are you an optimist or a pessimist? Do you make lemonade when life gives you lemons? When you get to the end of your rope, do you tie a knot and hang on? Do you see the rose and not the thorns or do you stare at the thorns, oblivious to the rose?

Have you heard the expression attributed to Harry S. Truman, "A pessimist is one who makes difficulties of his opportunities, and an optimist is one who makes opportunities out of his difficulties?" Glass half-full thinking implies that you have hope for a good outcome, and you dwell on the hopeful aspects of a situation. It doesn't mean that you never have a negative thought or feel down or disappointed. And it doesn't mean you don't allow yourself to feel your emotions.

Although we all need to experience our full range of emotions, glass half-full thinking means believing that something good or an invaluable lesson will come out of every situation. You will become more positive, confident, and eventually find peace and contentment because of this hope.

In her book, *Emotional Agility,* Susan David describes emotional agility as a process that enables us to navigate life's twists and turns with self-acceptance, clear-sightedness, and an open mind. The process isn't about ignoring difficult emotions and thoughts. It's about holding those emotions and thoughts loosely, facing them courageously and compassionately, and then moving past them to ignite change in your life.

There's a legend about two wolves that is often attributed to the Cherokee tribe: A grandfather is talking with his grandson, and he says there are two wolves inside of us which are always at war with each other. One of them is a good wolf which stands for things like kindness, bravery, and love. The other is a bad wolf, which stands for things like greed, hatred, and fear. The grandson stops and thinks about it for a second, then he looks up at his grandfather and says, "Grandfather, which one wins?" The grandfather quietly replies, "The one you feed."

Life is challenging for us all. If we ponder and meditate on the positive instead of the negative, we will begin to see the glass as half-full – this is half-full thinking.

Dig Deeper
Reflection and action:

1. Are you an optimist, a pessimist, or somewhere in-between?

2. This week, notice your reaction to things that happen. How do they make you feel?

3. Write down 3 things you will do to add more optimism in your life.

Resources and reading:

1. David, S. (2016). Emotional agility: Get unstuck, embrace change, and thrive in work and life. Avery.

TIP 4 - EAT "PLATE HALF-FULL"

"The doctor of the future will no longer treat the human frame with drugs, but rather will cure and prevent disease with nutrition."

Thomas A. Edison, inventor and businessman

The "plate method" for nutrition education has been around for many years but was catapulted into the spotlight by the food icon released in 2011 by the United States Department of Agriculture. This icon, called "MyPlate," replaced the food guide pyramid with a graphic illustration of a plate sectioned with components of a meal filled with healthy eating ideas. MyPlate recommendations are based on the Dietary Guidelines for Americans (DGA), which is published every five years by the United States Departments of Agriculture and Health and Human Services. The latest guidelines, released for 2020-2025, simplify important nutrition concepts into digestible bites with a focus on disease prevention and health promotion. This latest edition marks the first time the DGAs made recommendations by life stages, from birth through older adulthood. The theme is "Make every bite count with the Dietary Guidelines for Americans."

Do you make every bite count? Nutrition matters at every life stage. It's never too early or too late to eat healthfully. Begin now. If you get off track, get back on track at your next meal. There's no need to wait for the next day or the next week. Every day presents opportunities to nourish yourself. It's never too early to begin and it's never too late to start.

Some key recommendations from the guidelines for adults include:

1. Keep your nutrition needs in mind when you choose what to eat. Eat to meet nutrient needs, achieve a healthy body weight, and reduce the risk of chronic disease.

2. Your personal preferences, cultural traditions, and budget matter when choosing your healthy dietary pattern.

3. Focus on meeting food group needs with nutrient-dense foods and beverages. Nutrient-dense foods are foods that supply vitamins, minerals, and other health-promoting components and have no or little added sugars, saturated fat, and sodium.

You might sometimes hear these foods being called "whole" foods, or "real" foods, or "natural" foods, but these terms are not well-defined. According to the Academy of Nutrition and Dietetics, the terms "whole" or "natural" are not regulated terms, therefore, they don't have formal definitions. In general, the Food and Drug Administration (FDA) has considered the term natural to mean that nothing artificial or synthetic has been included or added to a food. And whole refers to foods not processed or refined.

Like the DGAs, I prefer the term nutrient-dense or nutrient-rich. A healthy dietary pattern consists of nutrient-dense forms of foods and beverages across all food groups, in recommended amounts, and within calorie limits. While I don't encourage most people to get caught up in counting calories, there are some useful resources from MyPlate.gov that can help you get a general idea about how much to include on your plate. But for a thorough assessment and help with questions about how much to eat, my best advice is to work with a registered dietitian nutritionist (RDN). More on that in Tip 6 – Feel Great and Love Your Plate – and Tip 17 – You Are You-nique.

The core elements that make up a healthy eating plan or dietary pattern include:

• vegetables of all types - dark green, red, and orange, beans, peas, lentils, and starchy and non-starchy vegetables

• fruit- including fresh, frozen, canned, or dried without added sugar, and 100% fruit juice in limited amounts (4 ounce or less per day)

• grains - at least half of which are whole grain, including bread, pasta, quinoa, rice, and cereal

• dairy - including fat-free or low-fat milk, yogurt, cheese, including lactose-free versions, and fortified soy beverages and soy yogurt alternatives

• protein foods - including lean meats, poultry, eggs, seafood, beans, peas, lentils, nuts, seeds, and soy products (e.g., tempeh and tofu)

• oils - including vegetable oils and oils in food, such as seafood and nuts

Also included in the DGAs are recommended limits for saturated and trans fats (less than 10% of calories), added sugars (less than 10% of calories – more on this subject in Tip 41), sodium (less than 2300 mg per day), and alcohol (If alcohol is consumed, it should be consumed in moderation – up to one drink per day for women and up to two drinks per day for men – and only by adults of legal drinking age).

The importance of physical activity is highlighted in the DGAs because of the role physical activity or exercise plays in promoting health and reducing the risk of developing chronic disease. Diet and exercise go hand in hand as the two main parts of the calorie balance equation to help manage body weight. For adults, the Physical Activity Guidelines for Americans include at least 150-300 minutes of moderate-intensity aerobic activity, like brisk walking or fast dancing, each week. Adults also need muscle-strengthening activity, like lifting weights, at least 2 days each week.

So, what is "plate half-full" and why is this important? Let's turn our attention to the vegetable and fruit part on the plate. According to the USDA MyPlate recommendations, your plate should be half full of vegetables and fruits.

This is one of my most important pieces of advice: first, fill half your plate with vegetables or vegetables and fruits.

According to the National Health and Nutrition Examination Survey (NHANES), a program of the Centers for Disease Control and Prevention, only 1 in 10 Americans eat the recommended servings per day of vegetables and fruits. That means 90% of adult Americans are falling below the recommendations of 1½ - 2 cups per day of fruits and 2 - 3 cups per day of vegetables. Surely, there's work to be done, and a wonderful place to start is to fill half your plate with vegetables and fruits.

The Wegmans supermarket chain was ahead of the USDA with their "half-plate healthy" campaign. As explained by Krystal Register, the former RDN for Wegmans' Virginia and Maryland stores, "We, at Wegmans, recommend that you fill half your plate with fruits and vegetables and the other half with anything else." Register explained this at a medical professionals' sneak peek tour, "Based on research, if people fill half of their plates with vegetables and fruits, then they make healthier choices for the other half."

We can all look at our plates at each meal and see if half of our plate is filled with vegetables or vegetables and fruits. We can do this. We can. You can!

Dig Deeper

Reflection and action:

1. Fill half your plate with vegetables, or vegetables and fruits for at least one meal per day, then increase to two meals per day and,

finally, three meals per day by the end of the week.

Resources and reading:

1. U.S. Department of Agriculture and U.S. Department of Health and Human Services. *Dietary Guidelines for Americans, 2020-2025*. 9th Edition. December 2020. Available at https://www.dietaryguidelines.gov/resources/2020-2025-dietary-guidelines-online-materials

2. Physical Activity Guidelines for Americans - https://health.gov/our-work/nutrition-physical-activity/physical-activity-guidelines/current-guidelines

3. Food Marketing Terms - https://www.eatright.org/food/nutrition/nutrition-facts-and-food-labels/understanding-food-marketing-terms

4. How much to include on your plate - https://www.myplate.gov/myplate-plan

5. Centers for Disease Prevention and Control Newsroom. *Only 1 in 10 adults get enough fruits or vegetables.* https://www.cdc.gov/media/releases/2017/p1116-fruit-vegetable-consumption.html

TIP 5 - LIVE A FULL LIFE

"Health and cheerfulness naturally beget each other."

Joseph Addison, English essayist

Put 'half-full' thinking together with "half-plate" eating, and I believe it will help you to move towards living a full life. In other words, optimistic thinking together with healthy eating leads to fullness in life. Imagine it as a formula for a healthy life:

Glass half-full thinking + plate half full of vegetables
and fruits = fullness in eating

Optimistic thinking + healthy eating = fullness in life

Clearly, nobody knows for sure how long we will live. In fact, one of the biggest arguments that I've been met with my whole career is, "So and so ate healthy and still died early, so why bother? I want to enjoy life and eat what I want." My response is, "Perhaps the most important thing isn't just about adding years to your life. It's about adding life to your years."

We want to be fully alive while physically alive - to live a full life.

I love the research by Dan Buettner, a National Geographic Fellow, Blue Zones researcher, and author. The Blue Zones are areas in the world where people live both the longest and healthiest lives. Regions include Ikaria (Greece), Sardinia (Italy), Okinawa (Japan), Nicoya Peninsula (Costa Rica), and Loma Linda (California). We have much to learn from people in the Blue Zones.

<u>Dig Deeper</u>

Reflection and action:

1. Write down what it means to you to be fully alive.

2. Write down steps you want to take, beginning this week, to add life to your years.

Resources and reading:

1. Buettner, D. (2012). *The blue zones: second edition: 9 lessons for living longer from the people who've lived the longest.* National Geographic.

2. Salmansohn, K. (2018). *Life is long: 50+ ways to help you live a little bit closer to forever.* 10 Speed Press.

3. Salmansohn, K. (2020). *Happy habits: 50 science-backed rituals to adopt (or stop) to boost health and happiness.* 10 Speed Press.

TIP 6 - FEEL GREAT AND LOVE
YOUR WEIGHT

"The curious paradox is that when I accept myself
just as I am, then I can change."

Carl Rogers, psychologist

L ove your weight? Yes, love your weight!! I can hear the murmurs, snickers, and maybe even grumbling now. Who loves their weight?

After interviewing thousands of people, I can answer that question: not very many! I can say, with confidence, that people who love their weight are in the minority. But self-acceptance is a doorway to change, just as Carl Rogers expressed in the above quote.

"Love your neighbor as yourself" is considered one of the greatest commandments given by God, according to Jesus in the Gospel of Mark. Most people realize they need to work on "loving their neighbor," but underestimate the importance of loving themselves. Remember, you can't pour from an empty cup.

Are you your worst critic? Do you listen to that inner voice that is often accusing or judgmental? To move forward with self-care and self-improvement, we need to recognize that self-acceptance matters, too.

Maya Angelou said, "Do the best you can until you know better, and then when you know better, do better." Don't beat yourself up for things you might have believed in the past that you don't believe now. It's good to change your mind for the better. That's what self-improvement is all about. Strive to be a better person than you were yesterday. That's the only comparison worth making.

So, how does weight fit into this thinking? If your blood

pressure is within the healthy range, and your lab work is within normal healthy ranges, and you are comfortable in your own skin, then you already may be loving your weight. Lab work may include blood sugar, hemoglobin A1C, blood lipids, such as cholesterol, LDL and HDL cholesterol, triglycerides, and liver enzymes, among others. But many people, including most of the clients I've worked with over the years, do not feel this way at the beginning of their health journey.

How do you get to the place of loving your weight, especially when you want to lose weight? If you feel like you need help getting started, working with a registered dietitian nutritionist (RDN) can help immensely. RDNs provide individualized advice, also called medical nutrition therapy, for your unique nutrition needs and medical conditions. Seeking nutrition advice can be confusing. Anyone can call themselves a nutritionist, but an RDN must meet strict criteria, including earning at least a four-year degree from an accredited nutrition curriculum, completing an extensive supervised program of practice, passing a rigorous registration exam, and maintaining annual continuing education credits.

The Academy of Nutrition and Dietetics' *Find a Nutrition Expert* allows you to search a national database to help you find an RDN in your area (see resources and reading).

You have probably already discovered that losing weight is one thing and keeping it off is quite another. Some people think that losing weight is the easy part and keeping it off is the hard part. Both are challenging. There are no quick fixes, despite the many advertisements promoting them.

There are a lot of different statistics about the rates of successful weight loss and weight maintenance. I'm not a huge fan of these statistics because I've worked with enough people to know that statistics don't necessarily motivate most people to change. In fact, some can be downright discouraging. There are so many variables to consider when looking at studies about weight loss or weight maintenance, including the age and sex of participants and the amount of weight lost. The following questions also need to be considered or answered: Were participants working with an RDN? Were they following safe weight loss guidelines or going to extreme fad diet measures? Was the study over six months, one year, two years, or five years? And there are other variables, too.

According to the Centers for Disease Control and Prevention, even a modest weight loss of 5-10% of your total body weight is likely to produce health benefits, such as improvements in blood pressure, blood cholesterol, and blood sugar. For example, if you weigh 200 pounds, that would be a weight loss of 10-20 pounds. This is the best place to start. I have found this is achievable.

But what does this have to do with loving your weight? A lot! Remember, self-acceptance is the doorway to change. Even if you are already at a weight where you are enjoying great health and lab work, loving your weight is not a given. I know many people who are at a healthy weight and still struggle with loving their weight or body acceptance.

Here are some tips, shared from the National Eating Disorders Association website, that will help you begin to better appreciate and love your weight:

1. Create a list of all the things your body lets you do. Read it and add to it often.
2. Wear comfortable clothes that you like, that express your personal style, and that feel good to your body.
3. Be your body's friend and supporter, not its enemy.
4. Consider this: your skin replaces itself once a month, your stomach lining every five days, your liver every six weeks, and your skeleton every three months. Your body is extraordinary—begin to respect and love it.
5. Every evening when you go to bed, tell your body how much you appreciate what it has allowed you to do throughout the day.

Dig Deeper

Reflection and action:

1. Create your own list of the things your body lets you do. For example, my body helps me work and accomplish my dreams. My body helps me dance and sing when I'm happy. My body helps me digest the food I eat so I am well-nourished and have energy. Read it and add to it often.

Resources and reading:

1. The Academy of Nutrition and Dietetics. Find a Nutrition Expert in your area - https://www.eatright.org/find-an-expert

2. Eating Disorder Association (NEDA) - https://www.nationaleatingdisorders.org/

3. 20 Ways to Love Your Body compiled by Margo Maine on NEDA website – https://tinyurl.com/mpnvwr6d

4. Centers for Disease Control and Prevention. *Losing Weight.* https://www.cdc.gov/healthyweight/losing_weight/index.html

TIP 7 - NOURISH YOURSELF AND LIMIT ULTRA-PROCESSED FOODS

"If we could give every individual the right amount of nourishment and exercise, not too little and not too much, we would have found the safest way to health."
Hippocrates

"Cooking (from scratch) is the single most important thing we could do as a family to improve our health and general well-being."
Michael Pollan, author

Most people eat to satisfy their hunger, not thinking much about nourishing their bodies. But our bodies need nourishment. We need nutrients. Over 40 nutrients have been identified as essential, meaning our bodies need them every day. We cannot make them ourselves. We need to consume them.

These include carbohydrates, protein (10 amino acids), fat (two essential fatty acids), water, vitamins (nine water-soluble and four fat-soluble) and 15 minerals. If we don't consume them in sufficient amounts, we will become nutrient-deficient, and our bodies won't work to the best of their abilities. So, while eating helps us to satisfy hunger, and supplies lots of enjoyment, it also nourishes us.

Since nutrition is a relatively young science, it makes sense that we don't currently know all that there is to know about it. According to a 2018 article in the *British Medical Journal*, "History of modern science – implications for current research, dietary guidelines, and food policy," the first vitamin was named in 1926, less than 100 years ago! And the role of nutrition in chronic diseases, such as heart disease, diabetes, and cancer, began in the past two to three decades, and mainly after 2000. Most likely, there are more nutrients to be discovered. It's a beautiful thing that food is made up of the nutrients we need, in the right proportions, in the right package. Food is our best source of the nutrients our bodies need.

So, the next time you're hungry, instead of just thinking about eating something that's handy and available, think about eating something to nourish every cell in your body. Eat foods that help you feel your best, think your best, move your best, and look your best!

We talked about nutrient-dense or nutrient-rich foods in Tip 4. I explained that nutrient-dense foods are foods that provide vitamins, minerals, and other health-promoting components and have no or little added sugars, fat, and sodium. This means that these foods are closer to their natural state without a lot of processing. On the other hand, energy-dense foods provide a high number of calories for the amount of food. Energy-dense equals calorie-dense. For example, blueberries are a nutrient-dense food and blueberry pie is an energy-dense food with added sugar, fat, and refined grains. Chicken breast is nutrient-dense. while breaded, deep-fried chicken breast is energy dense. Enjoy more nutrient-dense foods and less-energy dense foods.

In terms of hunger and fullness, the nutrient composition of a meal determines the extent to which food produces satiation and sustains satiety. Protein is the most satiating of the nutrients that supplies calories.

Satiating Foods
- Protein (such as fish, chicken, beef, dairy, eggs, nuts, and beans)

- Nutrient-dense foods (such as vegetables, fruits, whole grains, beans, and lean protein)

- High fiber foods (such as vegetables, fruits, whole grains, and beans)

You may think that foods high in fat are satisfying, but fat has a weak effect on satiation, so high fat foods may lead to overeating. Think about how easy it is to overeat potato chips or donuts. This is because the satiety signals are produced only after food enters the intestine. Fat in the intestine triggers the release of cholecystokinin – a hormone that signals satiety and inhibits food intake. So, this takes a while and people often overeat portions before the fullness is felt.

You may think that high sugar foods help ease your hunger, but the effects are short-lived. Once your blood sugar levels drop, hunger quickly returns. Sometimes people refer to this as a "sugar crash." If you're eating mostly refined carbohydrates and high sugar foods, you can feel like you're on a roller coaster going between high blood sugar levels after you eat and low blood sugar levels after the crash. Unfortunately, this is common.

Eating high-fat foods while trying to limit calorie intake, requires being aware of portions. Eating slowly and mindfully, helps with eating less of these foods and with eating less, in general.

Also, certain food combinations are more filling than others. Combining protein-rich foods such as fish, chicken, lean beef, dairy, and nuts with high fiber foods such as beans, whole grains, or vegetables and fruits, add staying power and help increase satiety. Foods that are high in water content, such as fruits and veggies, are nutrient-rich and contain fiber, helping to fill you up without a lot of calories. Other high fiber foods such as beans and whole grains are also nutrient-dense.

Another way to look at nutrient-dense foods versus energy-dense foods is to consider the processing of the foods. Since 2009, there's been a classification system looking at how food is processed. Recognized by the World Health Organization, it is called the NOVA classification. It was developed by Dr. Carlos Monteiro and his team at the Center for Epidemiological Research in Nutrition and Health at the University of Sao Paulo, Brazil.

The NOVA system classifies foods into four categories:

- Group 1 - Unprocessed or minimally processed foods
- Group 2 - Processed culinary ingredients
- Group 3 - Processed foods
- Group 4 - Ultra-processed food and drink products

A recent search on The National Library of Medicine at the National Institutes of Health's PubMed.gov, a free search engine accessing the Medline database of references and abstracts on the life sciences and biomedical topic, revealed over 700 papers with the term ultra-processed food. Hopefully, this topic will receive more attention in the future.

According to the NOVA classification groups, unprocessed or minimally processed foods include the natural edible food parts of plants and animals. They may be slightly altered for the main purpose of preservation but does not substantially change the nutritional content of the food. Many fresh fruits, vegetables, whole grains, nuts, meats, and milk fall into this category. Processed culinary ingredients are food ingredients minimally processed, such as oils from plants, seeds, nuts, or flour and pasta formed from whole grains.

On the other hand, processed foods include foods from groups one and two, but that have added salt, sugar, or fats. Ultra-processed foods are foods from groups one, two, and three, that go beyond the addition of fat, salt, or sugar, to include artificial colors and flavors and preservatives that promote shelf stability, preserve texture, and increase palatability. Examples include sugary drinks, cookies, some crackers and chips, some breakfast cereals, some frozen dinners, and luncheon meats. These are often more energy-dense.

Remember, the goal is to consume more nutrient-dense foods and less energy-dense foods. All of this is well supported by research which shows that limiting ultra-processed food and drinks is better for your health; consuming more nutrient-dense foods is better for your health.

Increased intake of ultra-processed foods has been linked with overeating, weight gain, and obesity. Dr. Kevin D. Hall of the National Institute of Diabetes and Digestive and Kidney Diseases (NIDDK), part of the National Institutes of Health (NIH), found that an increase of ultra-processed foods is linked with increased intake of energy-dense foods, decreased intake of fiber, and weight gain. He is currently conducting more research on this topic.

Dig Deeper

Reflection and action:

1. Do you think about eating to satisfy your appetite without giving thought to nourishing yourself?

2. Make a commitment to fill your plate and glass with foods and drinks that nourish your body.

3. Pay attention to how many nutrient-dense foods you choose daily compared with how many energy-dense or ultra-processed foods you consume.

Resources and reading:

1. Rolls, B., & Hermann, M. (2012). *The Ultimate Volumetrics Diet: Smart, simple, science-based strategies for losing weight and keeping it off.* William Morrows Cookbooks.

2. Seale, S.A., Sherard, T., & Fleming, D. (2010). *The Full Plate Diet.* Bard Press.

TIP 8 - UNDERSTAND NORMAL EATING

"My doctor told me to stop having intimate dinners
for four, unless there are three other people."

Orson Welles, director, actor, screenwriter, and producer

I love the definition of normal eating originally described by Ellyn Satter, registered dietitian nutritionist, therapist, author, and lecturer. Her teachings have convinced me that she has the best definition of what normal eating is. Why would we even need a definition of normal eating? I believe it's because extremism in eating attitudes and habits lead many to become prisoners of what they think they "should" be eating. This results in great guilt associated with eating and deprives us of the joy of eating. No one is perfect, and there are no perfect eating habits. Perfection isn't the goal in healthy eating or in life. I love the expression that perfection is the enemy of progress. I tell my clients and myself, "choose progress over perfection."

According to Ellyn Satter:

- Normal eating is going to the table hungry and eating until you are satisfied.

- Normal eating is being able to choose food you like and eat it and truly get enough of it—not just stop eating because you think you should.

- Normal eating is being able to give some thought to your food selection so you get nutritious food, but not being so wary and restrictive that you miss enjoyable food.

- Normal eating is giving yourself permission to eat

sometimes because you are happy, sad, or bored, or just because it feels good.

- Normal eating is mostly three meals a day, or four or five, or it can be choosing to munch along the way.

- Normal eating is leaving some cookies on the plate because you know you can have some again tomorrow, or it is eating more now because they taste so wonderful.
- Normal eating is overeating at times and feeling stuffed and uncomfortable. And it can be under eating at times and wishing you had more.

- Normal eating is trusting your body to make up for your mistakes in eating.

- Normal eating takes up some of your time and attention but keeps its place as only one key area of your life.

- In short, normal eating is flexible. It varies in response to your hunger, your schedule, your proximity to food and your feelings.

Hopefully, you can identify with this definition of normal eating. If not, you're not alone. Many people today are out of touch with the basic feelings of hunger and fullness. Are you surprised that it's normal to occasionally overeat or under eat? Of course, we all do either at one time or another. But when either become a mindless habit, this may lead to imbalance and health issues. Being rigid about certain food rules can create extremism and stress when perfection isn't achieved.

Dig Deeper

Reflection and action:

1. Does this definition of "normal eating" sound like your relationship with eating?

2. Are there areas that could be improved in your thinking to help improve your relationship with food?

Resources and reading:

1. The definition of healthy eating is copyright as follows: Copyright 2016 by Ellyn Satter published at www.EllynSatterInstitute.org.

2. Satter, E. (2008). *Secrets of feeding a healthy family: How to eat, how to raise good eaters, 2nd edition.* Kelcy Press.

TIP 9 - PREVENTION IS THE BEST MEDICINE

"The doctor of the future will give no medication, but will interest his patients in the care of the human frame, diet and in the cause and prevention of disease."

Thomas A. Edison, inventor, and businessman

Preventing a lifetime of overeating begins in infancy. Babies instinctively know when to eat and when to stop. When a baby has had enough to eat or drink, he/she simply turns away expressing disinterest. Babies have a built-in awareness of hunger and fullness, and they honor this. But somewhere along the way, we all learn to override these feelings for one reason or another. When food tastes so good, do you keep on eating, even though you aren't truly hungry anymore? Did you learn to turn to food for comfort after experiencing pain? Did your mom give you a cookie when you fell and hurt yourself to console you? Did you ever bake a cake or eat ice cream when you had a rough day at school? Did you search the kitchen for something to eat when bored or stressed? Unfortunately, many are out of touch and unable to recognize basic feelings of hunger and fullness.

People often override their body's signals for fullness, and overeating becomes a way of life. Eventually, many people don't even notice their natural signals. They just stay over full and uncomfortable most of the time, or plough through the day without noticing productivity over self-care.

Parents who don't pay attention to their body's natural hunger and fullness cues model this behavior for their children. Then, the children learn to override their own natural signals and this unnatural behavior is reproduced. I have seen this happen with too many Americans over the course of my dietetics' practice.

According to the Centers for Disease Control and Prevention's (CDC) data, the prevalence of U.S. obesity reported in 2019 was 42.4%. This is up from 30.5% in 1999-2000. Obesity-related conditions include heart disease, stroke, type 2 diabetes, and certain types of cancer, which are some of the leading causes of preventable, premature death.

By paying better attention to our body's natural signals for hunger and fullness, we can improve health and reduce risk for developing these chronic diseases. And if you already have high blood pressure, type 2 diabetes, or heart disease, you can manage your symptoms and prevent complications. If you feel your fullness and say, "I'm full or I'm satisfied," instead of waiting until you feel overfull or stuffed, you will be mindful to prevent overeating. Learning to be satisfied with less will help you lose weight, if desired. It will help you enjoy your food more, feel better, and maintain a healthy weight.

Dig Deeper

Reflection and action:

1. What are your body's signals for hunger and fullness?

2. Keep a log of your hunger and fullness before and after eating for the next week.

Resources and reading:

1. For further reading on mindful eating, I recommend books by Dr. Susan Albers and her website: www.eatingmindfully.com.

2. Centers for Disease Control and Prevention - https://www.cdc.gov/nchs/products/databriefs/db360.htm

TIP 10 - HUNGER AND FULLNESS

*"The more you eat, the less flavor; the less
you eat, the more flavor."*

Chinese Proverb

The human brain is so fascinating. Have you ever heard about the hypothalamus? This is the part of the brain known as the control center because it gives and receives messages about energy intake, expenditure, and storage from other parts of the brain and from the mouth, gastrointestinal (GI) tract, and liver. These messages influence satiation, which helps to control meal size, satiety, and regulate meal frequency.

Dozens of GI hormones influence appetite and food intake. Here are some examples:

- amylin
- cholecystokinin (CCK)
- enterostatin
- ghrelin
- glucagon-like Peptide-1 (GLP-1)
- oxyntomodulin
- pancreatic polypeptide (PP)
- peptide YY (PYY)

An important brain chemical that plays a vital role is Neuropeptide Y – a chemical produced in the brain that stimulates appetite, diminishes energy expenditure, and increases fat storage. It's responsible for causing carbohydrate cravings, and also initiates eating, decreases energy expenditure, and increases fat storage.

You have probably heard of some of these hormones as they are in the news quite often. Research is being conducted to find out more about how these hormones work, how they are turned on or off, how they influence intake, and how they could be used to help prevent or manage obesity.

Once your stomach and small intestine are empty, GI hormones are activated. Endorphins, your brain's pleasure chemicals, are triggered by the smell, sight, or taste of foods, enhancing your desire for them. Then you seek food and start eating. How much you eat is influenced by many factors, including social situations, personal mindfulness, time of day, and abundance of food.

In summary, true physiological hunger works like this:
- your stomach is empty and there aren't nutrients in your small intestine
- hormones in your gastrointestinal tract are activated
- endorphins – your brain's pleasure chemicals – are triggered by smell, sight, or taste of foods
- after the food enters your digestive tract, nutrients in the small intestine stimulate hormones, such as cholecystokinin, that slow stomach emptying and signal fullness
- finally, nutrients enter the blood, signal the brain via nerves and hormones, and tell the brain they are available for immediate use and/or storage

This continues until nutrients dwindle and hunger develops again.

Some factors that influence hunger:
- presence or absence of nutrients in bloodstream
- size and composition of the preceding meal
- customary eating patterns
- climate (heat reduces intake; cold increases it)
- exercise
- hormones
- illnesses

Your stomach is ideally designed for food to be delivered in small batches. It empties in about 4 hours, which is why most people feel hungry after 4 hours, and why our meals are generally spaced about 4 hours apart.

Let's look at some words used to describe fullness:

- Satiation is the feeling of satisfaction and fullness that occurs during a meal and halts eating. Satiation determines how much food is consumed during a meal.

- Satiety is the feeling of satisfaction and fullness that occurs after a meal and inhibits eating until the next meal. Satiety determines how much time passes between meals.

- Satiation tells us to "stop eating" and satiety reminds us to "not start eating again."

Do these mechanisms always work, or can we override them? Why isn't this fool proof? If it was just a physiological issue, it would be, but it is also environmental and psychological as well.

Environmentally, many eat mindlessly, and most don't overeat because of hunger. Environmental cues may trigger us to overeat. Some include being with family and friends, extra-large servings, and plates, enticing names, labels, and delicious smells.

Psychologically, I believe many also overeat because they look for satisfaction in food, rather than finding satisfaction elsewhere. Many overeat because they simply aren't paying attention. Many overeat because they are not being proactive TO NOT overeat. Overeating is quite easy! Not overeating requires thought. As someone once famously said, "Sometimes I sits and thinks and sometimes I just sits."

Autopilot doesn't help us achieve our goals. According to Dr. Wansink's research at the Cornell Food and Brand Lab at Cornell University, people make over 200 food decisions a day, 6,000 eating decisions in a month and 72,000 food decisions each year. Wow, no wonder we sometimes get confused!

How do you know when you're full? With so many distractions interfering with our body's cues, which many have ignored for too long, how does one tell the signs of fullness? Since it takes at least 20 minutes for your brain to get the message of fullness, it is best to eat slowly so that you will be able to sense fullness while you're eating.

But many people are no longer able to sense these feelings or maybe they have never paid attention.

If we are full, we are satisfied and if we are satisfied, we're full. Therefore, I recommend eating until one is satisfied and full and not until one is overfull or stuffed. In the book *The Blue Zones Solution,* the Okinawans in Japan have an expression, "hara hachi bu" to describe this feeling. It is a teaching that recommends that people eat only until they are approximately 80% full. While I personally feel this is difficult to gauge, I like to practice eating until my hunger symptoms are no longer present and I feel good. In other words, my stomach isn't growling, the shakiness or fuzzy thinking is gone, and I'm feeling more energetic. This requires some skill and practice, and mindful eating every day. The more you practice, the better you will become. Every meal and snack offer an opportunity to improve your skills.

There are many examples of hunger and fullness scales available. Here is one to give you an idea. Basically, neutral is in the middle and signifies neither hunger nor fullness. I recommend trying to stay within 3-7 on the scale. Being too hungry triggers overeating and being too full promotes weight gain and lethargy.

An example of a hunger and fullness scale can be seen on the next page.

Hunger and Fullness Scale:

1 = extreme hunger, feeling like you are starving
2 = very hungry
3 = hungry
4 = stomach starting to growl
5 = neutral - no feelings of hunger or fullness
6 = almost satisfied
7 = full and satisfied
8 = very full
9 = stuffed
10 = sick from being overstuffed and overfull

Dig Deeper

Reflection and action:

1. How long do you go after a meal before you notice you are hungry again?

2. Do you notice changes in your appetite, based on the factors that influence hunger listed above?

3. Keep track of your hunger and fullness before and after every meal for the next week.

Resources and reading:

1. Tribole, E. & Resch, E. (2012). *Intuitive eating.* St. Martin's Griffin.

2. Whitney, E. & Rolfes, S.R. (2013). *Understanding nutrition.* Wadworth, Cengage Learning.

3. Wansink, B. (2014). *Slim by design: Mindless eating solutions for everyday life.* William Morrow.

TIP 11 - ARE YOU HUNGRY?

"Sometimes late-night food cravings just mean
that you should be going to bed earlier."

Author Unknown

Recognizing the difference between physical hunger and every other kind of emotional hunger can prevent over-eating and weight gain. Instead, you can find constructive ways to feel better without food. I will share many tips in Part 3 of this book.

Physical signs of hunger:
- growling or rumbles in your stomach
- slight headache or difficulty concentrating
- feeling grumpy or irritable
- develops gradually
- occurs several hours after eating
- goes away when full
- eating leads to satisfaction

Emotional hunger cues:
- emotionally charged event precipitates hunger
- feeling sad or lonely
- feeling bored
- craving certain foods
- may develop suddenly
- occurs anytime of the day or night
- persists despite feeling full
- eating leads to feelings of guilt and shame
- never satisfied

Environmental eating cues:
- candy dish on desk or counter
- food visible on kitchen counters
- size of plates and glasses – people subconsciously eat more when eating on larger plates and drink more from larger glasses (more on this later)
- cheaper prices for larger sizes
- generous portions in restaurants

So, how can you tell if you are truly hungry? Physical signs of hunger tend to come on gradually and can be satisfied with any number of foods. Emotional hunger comes on suddenly, seems urgent, causes specific food cravings, and isn't satisfied. It's best to find another skill to satisfy emotional hunger because it won't be satisfied by food. Part 3 of this book has many tips and tools to better manage stress without food.

Now that you know the differences between various hungers, it's important to check in with yourself when you think you're hungry to fully assess whether it's best to eat or choose another activity to help you feel your best. I encourage my clients to make a list of the top 5-10 favorite things they enjoy doing besides eating. Then, I recommend they choose something from this list when they want to eat but are not truly hungry.

It's important to note here that sometimes we are simply thirsty instead of hungry, so make sure you are staying hydrated throughout the day. Our bodies are over 60% water, and we must take in enough to keep our bodies functioning at their best. We will talk more about hydration in an upcoming tip.

We crave foods for many reasons, both physical and emotional. From my experience working with patients over the years, food cravings often seem to be the result of irregular eating patterns, not paying attention to hunger and fullness, and making poor food choices. As I stated, there are over 40 essential nutrients our bodies need. If we fill up on foods that give us calories and not nutrients, our bodies may continue to crave food, hoping to get those needed nutrients.

If honoring hunger and fullness is so important, why do so many ignore these important self-regulating signals? Here are some common reasons I've heard over the years:

- **Stress**
  Did you know desserts are stressed spelled backwards?

- **Boredom**
  I don't have anything else to do so I think I'll eat. This happens when you find yourself standing in front of an open fridge, wondering what to eat.

- **Time of day**
  Eating by the clock instead of by your body's signals

- **Availability of food**
  Someone offers you something, so you eat it even though you're not hungry. You grab candy from the candy jar at work or eat doughnuts because they are in the break room.

- **Sight of food**
  Many tell me they're on the "see-food" diet. I see food, I eat it.

- **Taste of food**
  I'm full but I keep eating because it tastes so good.

- **Generous portion sizes**
  Super-sized portions trigger overeating.

It may take a while to regain your ability to identify true hunger and fullness. If you continue to have problems, I recommend working with a registered dietitian nutritionist (RDN), the experts in nutrition.

Dig Deeper

Reflection and action:

1. What are your physical signs of hunger?

2. What are your emotional signs of hunger?

3. What are your environmental cues?

4. Do you ignore your self-regulating signals? If so, why?

5. List your top 5-10 favorite activities that you enjoy doing besides eating?

Resources and reading:

1. The Academy of Nutrition and Dietetics. Find a Nutrition Expert in your area - https://www.eatright.org/find-an-expert.

2. Wansink, B. (2014). *Slim by design: Mindless eating solutions for everyday life.* William Morrow.

TIP 12 - EAT REGULARLY – KNOW THE IMPORTANCE OF HABITS

"One cannot think well, love well, sleep
well, if one has not dined well."
Virginia Woolf, English author

"The single best investment you can make to your health on a
daily basis – in fact, at least three times a day – is to eat well."
Dr. Wendy Bazilian, nutrition/fitness expert and author

Many of my clients who come for help to lose weight are not even eating regularly. Every day is different for them; there's no consistency or order. This is one form of disordered eating. While every person is unique and has their own individual pattern that works best for them, having a consistent pattern matters.

Common problems and solutions are listed below:

Problem: "I don't have time to eat." Time for preparing food and eating is not even factored into the day. Just like any other appointment on your calendar, you should plan to take time to eat. It's an investment in your health, not a waste of time.

Solution: Plan at least 20-45 minutes per meal for at least 2-3 meals per day. If you only eat two major meals, plan at least one or two more nutritious snacks or mini meals.

Problem: "I feel sick if I eat in the morning." A lot of times this happens to people who eat too late into the night. Your body digests at night and you can wake up not feeling so great.

Solution: Don't eat a lot before bed. If you choose to eat an evening snack, have a light snack of 15 grams of carbohydrate and/ or 6-8 grams of protein. Some examples include a small bowl of cereal and milk, ½ peanut butter sandwich on whole grain bread, apple slices with peanut butter, or 1-2 small pieces of dark chocolate (70% or more cacao is best) with ½ cup milk or milk alternative. If you choose to eat an evening snack, it's best to eat at least 1-2 hours before bed.

Problem: "If I eat in the morning, I'm hungrier all day, but if I don't eat, I can go all day and that saves calories." Most people who experience this, are not choosing nutrient dense foods. Instead, they are choosing high sugar foods, such as sweet cereal, pop tarts, muffins, and doughnuts. These high carbohydrate, low protein, and low fiber foods raise blood sugar quickly and cause the blood sugar to crash later, leaving one feeling hungrier.

Solution: Include whole grains, protein, and fiber in your breakfast. A few examples include eggs, whole grain toast and fruit, Greek yogurt with fruit and nuts, whole grain, low sugar cereal with milk, fruit, and nuts. Many of my clients believe skipping breakfast saves calories, but this often isn't the case because your metabolism may compensate by slowing down and burning less calories, and it may trigger overeating later in the day to compensate.

Dig Deeper

Reflection and action:

1. Do you have an eating pattern that works well for you?

2. If not, what changes would you like to make?

Resources and reading:

1. Krieger, E. (2013). *Small changes, big results. Revised and updated edition.* Clarkson Potter.

TIP 13 - AVOID EXTREMES

"The spirit cannot endure the body when overfed, but, if underfed, the body cannot endure the spirit."

Saint Frances de Sales, Bishop of Geneva and author

Have you ever felt so ravenous that you thought you were going to pass out? And then after eating, you felt so stuffed that you needed to lie down? These are the extremes. Many eaters go from starving to stuffed on a regular basis.

Many of my clients skip breakfast because they are too tired to make it and too rushed to take time to eat it. Later at work, their busy schedules interfere with lunch. By the time they get home from work, they are feeling ravenous and begin to eat everything in sight. Often this continues until bedtime.

Bypassing your natural cues for hunger, such as stomach growling, and allowing yourself to get to the point where you feel like you are starving, triggers overeating. I've seen this thousands of times in my clients' lives and I've experienced it in my own life before I began to pay attention and be more mindful of my hunger and fullness.

Zeroing in on your body's cues can help you eat when hunger hasn't gotten too extreme and stop when you are satisfied. Saying those two simple words, "I'm full," can help you avoid the extremes and feel better. These words empower you to eat mindfully instead of mindlessly.

When you're either starving or stuffed, you're at extremes in the spectrum of hunger and fullness. And either of these extremes can be dangerous. When you let your body get to the place where you feel like you are starving, you've gone too long without eating. The usual result of that extreme hunger is overeating. This is one of the biggest problems I encounter.

When my kids were little, and they would tell me that they were starving, I would gently remind them that children who go without food for days are starving. "You're hungry," I would say, helping them to rightly name those feelings to avoid that extreme expression that sometimes justifies overeating or stuffing oneself.

Likewise, the feeling of being stuffed is a negative feeling, although many people don't see it that way. When I was younger, I ate until I was stuffed at most every meal. When I ask children how they know when to stop eating, they tell me "When I feel sick," or "when my belly hurts." This was very eye-opening when I began to work with children.

When you're feeling stuffed, you've eaten more than your body needs. If you eat more than your body needs on a regular basis, then you will gain weight, unless you step up your exercise to burn off the extra calories. Unfortunately, it is much quicker and easier to eat a couple of hundred calories than it is to burn off a couple of hundred calories.

Consider the following ways to add approximately 200 calories. Each of these items has about 200 calories:

- 19 potato chips
- 3 chocolate chip cookies
- 12 ounces cranberry juice
- 3.5 ounces of vanilla ice cream
- 2 tablespoons peanut butter
- 1 package Reese's cups

Consider approximately how much exercise is necessary to burn those calories. Each activity burns about 200 calories:

- 30 minutes swimming
- 30 minutes climbing stairs
- 45 minutes of walking
- 45 minutes gardening
- 60 minutes of housecleaning

Dig Deeper

Reflection and action:

1. Continue to keep track of your hunger and fullness before and after meals.

2. Are you avoiding the extremes of hunger and fullness?

TIP 14 - UNDERSTAND THE POWERFUL 20

"Pace, don't race."

Susan Albers, Psy.D., clinical psychologist and author

Satiety is the feeling of satisfaction that occurs after a meal that inhibits eating until the next meal. When it comes to satiety or feeling your fullness, the power of 20 minutes rules! It takes about 20 minutes to sense fullness so it's important to eat slowly and pay attention to your signals. It's up to each of us to be mindful, conscientious eaters who sharpen our own awareness of hunger and fullness.

In addition to following the 80% rule mentioned in Tip 10, saying grace or giving thanks before meals helps you focus on gratitude for the food you are about to eat, as well as serving as a reminder to eat mindfully. Use a hunger and fullness scale, such as the one in Tip 10, to rate your level of fullness after you finish a meal.

In their book *Intuitive Eating,* Evelyn Tribole and Elyse Resch point out that the longer you have been disconnected from your body's sense of fullness, the longer it will take to identify fullness. A few tips they offer to increase your consciousness of fullness include:

- Eat without distraction to help you enjoy your eating experience and focus on it.

- Reinforce your conscious decision to stop by putting your utensils down, or putting your napkin on your plate, or nudging your plate slightly forward.

- Defend yourself from obligatory eating by practicing saying, "No, thank you."

Taking at least 20 minutes to eat your meal is the best way to allow yourself to actually feel your fullness. For fast eaters, it helps to put your fork down between bites, enjoy more conversation, and chew foods thoroughly. And if it isn't possible to take 20 minutes to eat, take the time you have and make that quality time being mindful to savor the flavor of each bite, enjoy your meal, and know that you will not actually feel your fullness for 20 minutes.

Say "I'm full" to tell yourself and others that you have finished eating and don't want more.

Dig Deeper

Reflection and action:

1. How long does it usually take you to eat from the beginning of a meal to the end? Time yourself to see.

2. Be mindful to slow down and pace, don't race. Time yourself over the next week to see if you are allowing enough time to enjoy your meal and feel your fullness.

Resources and reading:

1. Tribole, E. & Resch, E. (2012). *Intuitive eating.* St. Martin's Griffin.

2. Buettner, D. (2012). *The blue zones, second edition: 9 lessons for living longer from the people who've lived the longest.* National Geographic Society.

TIP 15 - EAT MINDFULLY, NOT MINDLESSLY

"When walking, walk. When eating, eat."

Zen Proverb

"Eat slowly, with other people whenever possible,
and always with pleasure."

Michael Pollan, author

Most people eat mindlessly at one time or another. It seems to be the American way. Years ago, when research began emerging about the health benefits of the Mediterranean Diet, I had the feeling that these benefits were not only related to their diet, but also due to their lifestyle. Much research has shown this to be true. In those Blue Zones regions of the world (Tip 5), where people live the longest and healthiest lives, it is part of their respective cultures to eat mindfully.

Many Americans eat "on the way" to their next event, be it a meeting or sports event. In the Blue Zones and Mediterranean cultures, eating meals is more of a main event. Families and friends take time to plan, prepare and enjoy their food, and these practices contribute to healthier cultures and longer lives.

The Slow Food Movement began in Italy in 1986 as an alternative to fast food restaurants, which were popping up in their cities. Now, Slow Food is international and seeks to bring enjoyment of traditional and regional foods to all countries around the world. Many cities have local chapters where people enjoy meals together and promote education focused on the importance of slowing down and enjoying foods from many cultures.

In 2003, Susan Albers wrote the classic *Eating Mindfully*, and in 2007, Dr. Brian Wansink, wrote his classic *Mindless Eating.* In a recent search on the National Institutes of Health's website,

PubMed, 577 citations for articles about mindful eating attest to the interest in and research being conducted on the relationship between mindful eating and health.

Mindful eating changed my life. As I mentioned, I grew up overeating. Most every meal, I ate until all the food was gone and I was stuffed. This is why I'm passionate about this topic. I enjoy my food just as much now, but I feel better after meals and maintain my weight within a healthy range. After my counseling or classes, clients and participants tell me that they are satisfied with less food than previously. This is because they are paying more attention and realize that their appetites are satisfied with less food than they previously thought they needed. Paying attention and eating mindfully has improved their lives.

One simple way to improve awareness about eating mindfully is through a mindful eating exercise or meditation. I love doing this in my classes and with clients. It is always eye-opening and enjoyable. I recommend using a small piece of fruit, such as a grape or raisin, or a piece of dark chocolate. But any food will do. I've used dried cranberries, apple slices, mandarin orange sections, cherry tomatoes, to name a few.

Follow these steps and move very slowly through each one. Read the instructions the whole way through before beginning.

1. Look at the food as if you've never seen it before. Notice the colors, shapes, and texture. What do you notice about this food?

2. Smell the food and enjoy the aroma. Close your eyes. Do you have any food memories associated with this aroma?

3. Think about where and how the food was grown. Imagine the steps involved in growing this food or in bringing this food to you. Feel gratitude in your heart for the hands that produced this food.

4. Take a very small bite of the food, if using dark choc-

olate, but eat the full bite if you're using a small piece of fruit.

5. Instead of immediately chewing the food, move the bite of food around in your mouth and notice how it feels on your tongue. Is it cold, smooth, rough?

6. During the bite, you may want to close your eyes to shut out other stimulation and better notice the sensations of the food in your mouth.

7. Chew the food very slowly until it is a smooth texture. Chocolate melts at the temperature in your mouth, so you may not need to chew chocolate at all.

8. Swallow slowly and notice any aftertaste that lingers.

Dig Deeper

Reflection and action:

1. Most of the time, are you eating mindfully or mindlessly?

2. Complete the mindful eating exercise above.

3. How did eating the food slowly and mindfully influence the taste of the food?

4. How did eating slowly and mindfully affect your enjoyment of the food?

Resources and reading:

1. Albers, S. (2012). *Eating mindfully, 2nd Edition.* New Harbinger Publications.

2. The Slow Food Movement in the USA, visit www.slowfoodusa.org.

TIP 16 - SAVOR EVERY BITE

"Mindful eating is about awareness. When you eat mindfully, you slow down, pay attention to the food you're eating and savor every bite."

Susan Albers, PsyD, clinical psychologist and author

Years ago, I read a study showing that the greatest pleasure is derived from the first few bites of a food. After a few bites, taste buds start to lose their sensitivity to the natural flavors in food. As I began to eat more mindfully, I began to notice this for myself. Especially with sweets and rich, high calorie food. I began thinking, if it's true that the most pleasure comes from the first few bites, then why not stop with those first few bites? This was significant in helping me to enjoy a few bites of calorie-dense foods without overeating. It was an "ah-ha" moment; some foods are best enjoyed in a few small bites!

For example, when you eat a piece of cake, make it a small piece. Enjoy every bite. Savor it. Give yourself permission to enjoy it. Food was made to be enjoyed. The dieting mentality labels foods as good or bad. Unfortunately, this thinking often makes people feel good or bad depending on their food choices. I'm good when I choose good foods. I'm bad when I choose bad foods. This leads to guilt, shame, and remorse when eating food labeled as bad. When you learn to savor a few bites, you lose the guilt, shame, and remorse. You enjoy your food (and life) more fully.

It's not that you can never have a certain calorie-dense food you love, the key is twofold. First, how often do you eat this food? Second, how much do you eat when you eat it? For example, I love fried foods. I know they are calorie-dense and not the best for heart health or my digestion. So, I limit my intake of these. I eat them when I can share them with family and friends. I don't eat them very often and I don't eat much of them when I do.

Learning to be satisfied with a few bites of food higher in calories and lower in nutritional value (calorie-dense), such as sweets and fried food, is the secret to enjoying them. Eliminating these items completely may promote feelings of deprivation, leading some people to binge eating, especially if they consider them comfort food.

One of the many reasons that diets don't work for permanent weight loss and health is because they lead to feelings of deprivation. The joke is that the word diet has the word die in it! Many weight loss diets consist of lists of good foods and bad foods. Unless you're following a special diet for specific medical reasons, it is usually not necessary to totally give up certain foods. Moderation helps promote a healthy relationship with food.

Be mindful about what you eat daily and keep in the house on a regular basis. For example, sweet desserts are not a necessary part of everyday meals. Choose healthier desserts and snack options daily, such as fruit and Greek yogurt. Serve sweeter, calorie-dense options less often. The goal is to enjoy nutrient-dense food with the frequency and in the portion size that allows you to achieve your health goals.

Dig Deeper

Reflection and action:

1. Do you categorize food as good or bad?

2. Write down a few food items that you love but feel guilty when eating. Consider how often you eat them and how much. Could you adjust your frequency and portion to help you enjoy these foods and still achieve your health goals?

Resources and reading:

1. Kristeller, J. (2015). *The Joy of half a cookie.* ORION.

2. Albers, S. (2019). *Hanger management: Master your hunger and improve your mood, mind, and relationships.* Little, Brown Spark.

POEM - PORTION DISTORTION

* * *

Portion Distortion

By Theresa Yosuico Stahl

"Can you help me with my diet?" So many inquire.
"What changes can I make to stop my
weight from going higher?"

I'll tell you my opinion in the simplest way.
We have portion distortion in the U.S. of A.

Yes, we've become the supersized generation.
And as a result, decreased the health of our nation.

So please everyone, please, downsize your portions.
Our overeating habits have reached epic proportions.

We need to rethink always adding those fries
And eat more fruits and veggies, and drink water besides.

And exercise daily, and eat a variety
of portions appropriate to our body's satiety.

Be mindful, be aware, and enjoy every bite.
And say "I'm full" to help you stay feeling all right.

We will feel so much better if we don't overstuff.
And to this portion distortion say enough is enough!

PART TWO - TIPS TO IMPROVE EATING SKILLS

* * *

TIP 17 - YOU ARE YOU-NIQUE

"Today you are you. It is truer than true. There's
no one alive who is youer than YOU."

Dr. Seuss, author, animator, and filmmaker

No two sets of fingerprints are the same. Not even for identical twins. And while identical twins share the same DNA, research is showing they develop differences due to mutations in their DNA. We are all individuals. We are unique. You are unique.

DNA, or deoxyribonucleic acid, is a molecule that contains the biological instructions that make each species unique. DNA, along with the instructions it contains, is passed from adult organisms to their offspring during reproduction.

Genetic testing has allowed us to learn about our personal DNA and our uniqueness. And personalized medicine, based on insights into your genes, is an emerging area of medicine.

Because we are all different, it's best to exercise caution when comparing ourselves with others. What works for you, may not work for me, and what works for me, may not work for you. For example, I am lactose intolerant. I lack the enzyme lactase, which helps to digest the milk sugar lactose, which is found in milk and many dairy products. If I drink cow's milk, I will experience gas, bloating, and possibly diarrhea. I prefer to drink soy or almond milk. If I told you that you needed to drink soy or almond milk, based on my own food intolerance, that wouldn't be good advice for you.

Doctors David and Catherine Katz have said, "Love the food that loves you back." In other words, love food and drink that make you feel good. Only you know which foods make you feel good and which ones don't, so only you know which ones love you back. Sticking with the lactose intolerance example, I love milk, but it doesn't love me back. So, I choose to drink an alternative to milk, such as soy or almond milk, or Lactaid milk, which has lactase enzyme added to it. Another personal example is eggs. I ate eggs most of my life, but I developed an intolerance to them after I had my gallbladder removed. Since our food intolerances may change throughout our lives, I hope that I will be able to tolerate them again.

Self-discovery in all areas is important work. Discovering your food intolerances, or the food that loves you back, is part of your journey of self-discovery. Always be a student of yourself. Listen to your body. Pay attention. Be mindful.

Sometimes, when someone discovers that certain food makes them sick, they may be inspired to inform others that these foods are bad for everyone, and, therefore, should be excluded from your diet. They write books and do the talk show or podcast circuit. But what they are saying is not necessarily true for you, just like me telling you not to consume milk or dairy products because of my own lactose intolerance. Our food intolerances are different. Our food preferences are different, too.

Our differences are in our genes which is why the advice to "love the food that loves you back" is so profound. You need to be the researcher of you. You are the best person for the job.

Slow down, pay attention, be mindful, and you will figure out which foods help you feel your best. Yes, there's evidence-based research about foods and nutrients and why balance, variety, and moderation matter. I strongly believe nutrition is a science. Tip 4 discusses the Dietary Guidelines for Americans. These are general guidelines. Michael Pollan distilled research regarding a general, healthy way to eat down to, "Eat food. Mostly plants. Not too much."

For individualized nutrition advice, called medical nutrition therapy, for your unique nutrition needs, check out the registered dietitian nutritionist (RDN) online referral service to help you find an RDN in your area (see resources and reading).

Dig Deeper

Reflection and action:

1. Have you ever kept a food log with a focus on how you feel after you eat? This week, keep track of your food and beverage intake along with symptoms such as energy levels, bloating, gas, bowel habits (normal, constipation, diarrhea), blood pressure levels, or blood sugar levels, if you have diabetes. Do any of your symptoms relate to your food intake? If you are working with an RDN, take this food and symptom log to your next appointment for review.

2. Have you been comparing your eating habits with others? Resolve to be a student of your own eating habits and resolve to stop comparisons.

Resources and reading:

1. Archibald, A. (2019). *The genomic kitchen.* Amanda Archibald.

2. The Academy of Nutrition and Dietetics. Find a Nutrition Expert in your area - https://www.eatright.org/find-an-expert

TIP 18 - FINDING COMMON GROUND

"Food is our common ground. Our universal experience."

James Beard, American chef and cookbook author

Does it sometimes seem like nutrition and medical professionals disagree more than they agree? This can be head-spinning, even for professionals. I even wrote a poem about my feelings about all the disagreements. I've included that poem, The Diet Riot, at the end of this section.

In 2015, the Oldways Finding Common Ground Conference brought a group of leading nutrition and food system experts together to reach consensus on common ground about healthy eating. Oldways is a nonprofit organization dedicated to improving public health. Their mission is to inspire individuals and organizations to embrace the healthy, sustainable joys of the "old ways" of eating – heritage-based diets high in taste, nourishment, sustainability, and joy.

Dissention seems more prevalent these days. Not just in differences about eating and food choices. We see the divides all around us. At this point in my life, I find inner peace and agreement more important than arguing, so I love finding common ground, when possible.

For over three decades in the nutrition world, I have seen the best evidence-based science change and evolve. Take eggs for example. When I first became an RDN, the National Cholesterol Education Program was new. The link between blood cholesterol levels and heart disease was changing nutrition education. Because egg yolks contained a high amount of cholesterol, nutrition recommendations were to limit egg yolks to three per week. Egg whites became popular. We advised substituting two egg whites for one egg in recipes.

Today, new ways to measure cholesterol in eggs, and new feeding practices of hens, have resulted in less cholesterol in eggs; almost 100 milligrams less per egg. In addition, research has shown that the amount of saturated fat in our diet influences blood cholesterol levels and heart disease risk more than the amount of dietary cholesterol. Consequently, even the American Heart Association now says consuming one egg per day can be part of a heart-healthy diet.

We see that nutrition research and nutrition guidelines evolve and change, based on the best available scientific evidence. That's why it's important to follow science.

Here are some of the common-ground recommendations that resulted from the Oldways Conference:

1. Eat more plants, nuts, legumes, and seafood.

2. Sustainability is essential. This means food security matters now and in the future. It's imperative to meet the food needs of the present without compromising the ability of future generations to meet their needs.

3. Food can and should be good times 3 – good for human health, good for the planet, and good as in unapologetically delicious.

4. Common ground in healthy eating should be promoted instead of confusion.

5. Healthy eating guidelines should be based on solid evidence.

6. Sensationalism should be avoided.

7. Recommendations for dietary changes should be meaningful, and practical dietary substitutions should be made.

8. Food literacy should be cultivated, believing that individuals benefit from knowing about the origins of

their food, the conditions under which it is produced, and its impact on their health and the health of the planet.

9. Food systems (food production to food waste) should align with priorities for human and planetary health while supporting social responsibility, justice, and animal welfare.

The full Oldways' consensus statement can be found at the link in the Dig Deeper section. For more information about food systems, and for inspiration about how you can help improve your local food system, check out the books *Stand Together or Starve Alone* and *Food Town USA* by author Mark Winne.

Dig Deeper

Reflection and action:

1. Notice sensational nutrition-related headlines and attention-grabbing titles that promote controversy and division.

2. Add more plants, nuts, legumes, and seafood in your daily meals and snacks.

3. Get involved in improving your food system. Do you have a food policy council in your area? If so, attend a meeting or food conference.

Resources and reading:

1. Oldways website – www.oldwayspt.org

2. Oldways Common Ground Consensus Statement on Healthy Eating – https://oldwayspt.org/programs/oldways-common-ground/oldways-common-ground-consensus

3. Winne, M. (2017). *Stand together or starve alone: Unity and*

chaos in the U.S. food movement. Praeger.

4. Winne, M. (2019). *Food town USA: Seven unlikely cities that are changing the way we eat.* Island Press.

TIP 19 - COMMON GROUND IN EATING FOR LONGEVITY AND BRAIN HEALTH

"May you live a long life full of gladness and health."

Irish Blessing

One of my favorite topics is eating for longevity and brain health. Maybe it's because I'm getting older and maybe it's because I love learning about how and why many people live long and healthy lives. This is exactly what numerous researchers have been doing over the past decade.

According to the Blue Zones series, five regions of the world that have the largest number of centenarians (people who live to at least 100 years-old): Loma Linda, California; Okinawa, Japan; Nicoya Peninsula, Costa Rica; and the Mediterranean regions of Sardinia, Italy, and Ikaria, Greece.

The Mediterranean Diet was selected by U.S. News and World Report's 2022 rankings as the top or tied for the top in the categories of best overall diet, best diet for heart disease, and best diet for diabetes. Heart disease and diabetes are in the top eight causes of death, according to the Centers for Disease Control and Prevention.

Some foods that stand out as promoting long, healthy lives and brain health include:

- avocados
- olive oil
- fish
- leafy green vegetables and other vegetables
- herbs and spices
- fruit
- beans, peanuts, and seeds

- yogurt and fermented foods
- whole grains

Some practical tips to get you started:

- Eat lots of vegetables. Make veggies the "stars" of the meal. Include dishes like Caprese salad, Greek salad, greens sauteed with garlic and olive oil, soups and stews, veggie-topped pizzas, and oven-roasted vegetables.

- Flavor with herbs, spices, and garlic, instead of salt. Grow your own herbs. When they are ready for harvest, I like to air dry mine, or dry in the oven, or puree with a little olive oil or water and freeze in ice cube trays.

- Use heart-healthy fats. Include sources of healthy fats in daily meals, especially extra-virgin olive oil, nuts, sunflower seeds, olives, and avocados. Substitute olive oil for butter – ¾ teaspoon for 1 teaspoon. There are blends of olive oil and butter on the market, for when you want butter.

- Eat meat as flavoring. Cook small strips of meat in a vegetable sauté, stir-fry, or add small amounts to pasta, salad, or soups. A little goes a long way.

- Enjoy dairy in moderation. Fermented dairy products, such as Greek yogurt and kefir are used more frequently in the Blue Zones, along with lesser amounts of a variety of flavorful cheeses, including goat and sheep's milk cheeses. Plain yogurt makes a great substitute for sour cream. For mayonnaise, try a substitute of 2/3 yogurt and 1/3 mayonnaise.

- Eat seafood twice a week. This is recommended by the American Heart Association, too. Fish such as tuna, herring, salmon, and sardines are rich in omega-3 fatty acids, and shellfish including mussels, oysters, and clams have similar benefits for brain and heart health.

- Cook more vegetarian meals. Build meals around beans, whole grains, and vegetables. Flavor with herbs and spices, which give added health benefits for brain health and longevity. For vegetarian re-cipe ideas, check out the Meatless Monday website at meatlessmonday.com.

- Eat more beans and lentils. Add these to soups and salads. Try roasting chickpeas for a simple snack. Simply rinse canned chickpeas and pat dry with a paper towel, spray with olive oil spray, and season to your taste with Mexican, Cajun, or Zaatar seasoning blend. Roast in the oven at 375 degrees Fahrenheit. until brown, about 30–45 minutes and shake them around on the pan every 15 minutes. Simple and flavorful. Include hummus as a snack or dip with raw veggies.

- Switch to whole grains, which are nutrient-rich, fla-vorful, and help you to feel full longer. Traditional Mediterranean grains include bulgur, barley, farro, and brown, black, or red rice.

- Eat fruit daily with meals or as snacks. Fruit is per-fect for dessert. It's sweet, light, and refreshing. Make smoothies with yogurt and fruit. Instead of a daily ice cream or cookies, have these sweets less frequently, and include fruit daily.

Dig Deeper

Reflection and action:

1. Are you including the foods listed above that help promote longevity and brain health?

2. This week, choose at least one of the tips above to implement daily.

Resources and reading:

1. Beuttner, D. (2017). *Blue zones solution.* National Geographic, 2017.

2. Linja, S.S. & Safaii-Waite, S. (2017). *The Alzheimer's prevention food guide.* Rockridge Press.

3. Moon, M. (2016). *The mind diet.* Ulysses Press.

4. Moon, M. (2019). *The telomere diet and cookbook* by Maggie Moon. Ulysses Press.

5. Raffetto, M. & Peterson, W.J. (2017). *Mediterranean diet cookbook for dummies.* For Dummies.

6. Patel, G. (2011). *Blending science with spices.* Feeding Health.

7. Blatner, D.J. (2010). *The flexitarian diet: The mostly vegetarian way to lose weight, be healthier, prevent disease, and add years to your life.* McGraw-Hill Education.

8. Salmansohn, K. (2018). *Life is long.* Ten Speed Press.

TIP 20 - DO YOU NEED A
TASTE BUD REHAB?

"I'm not telling you it's going to be easy - I'm telling
you it's going to be worth it."

Art Williams, insurance executive

What is the first thing that comes to your mind when you read or hear about rehab? Is it alcohol or drug rehab, or rehab that includes physical or occupational therapy? I first heard the words "taste bud rehab" from Dr. David Katz, lifestyle medicine physician, founding director of the Yale-Griffin Prevention Research Center at Yale University, and author. Those words, "taste bud rehab" stuck. This is something I've experienced first-hand in my life and what I've taught for years, but I never put it into those three words before hearing them from Dr. Katz.

Back in 1978, as a student at Western Maryland College, I took a psychology class and learned that it takes about 30 days to break a habit. More recent research on this topic has revealed a variety of magic-number-of-days to break a habit, anywhere from 21 to 254 days, unbelievably. But on average, current belief is that it takes about 60 days. For me, I took the 30 days I was taught in my class. I became addicted to ice cream shortly after arriving on the campus of Western Maryland College (now McDaniel College). After my lifetime of delicious, flavorful home-cooking, the college cafeteria food left much to be desired. All except the daily homemade rolls and hand dipped ice cream including eight flavors! This was heaven to an ice cream lover like me. As if this wasn't enough, just over the hill from the college was the best fruit stand/homemade ice cream shop. The freshman 15-plus became a reality in my life. Easy access, easy eating, and easy addiction.

I decided to give the "30 days to break a habit" rule a try. I went off ice cream "cold turkey," and lo and behold, it worked. I broke my daily craving for ice cream and my daily habit. While I still loved ice cream, I didn't have that "I need to eat ice cream every single day" desire. And hence, my first experience with taste bud rehab was born.

I always had a feeling that we crave what we eat. The more we eat something, the more we want it. My ice cream experience taught me that. I've noticed that people who drink sodas, crave sodas, while people that eat salads, crave salads. There is some science to back up my theory.

We have trillions of bacteria on and in us. These bacteria have been found to be critically important in many areas of health, especially the bacteria in our gut, that makes up what is called our gut microbiome. They have roles in digestion, nutrient absorption, and immune function, to name a few. Researchers at the National Institutes of Health's Human Microbiome Project have identified that the types of bacteria in our intestines are influenced by what we eat.

Could it possibly be that the more sweets we eat, the more sweet-loving gut bacteria we make? The more vegetables and fruits we eat, the more veggie and fruit loving gut bacteria we produce? What role does our gut bacteria play in the foods we love? Could it be that "the gut bacteria made me do it?" These are fascinating topics for further research.

All I know is that people who come to me with daily diets high in sugar crave sweets! Although they may like vegetables and fruits, they are eating only a minimum, if any. Throughout the course of several months of counseling or classes, dietary changes are made. Instead of drinking soda or sweet tea, they begin drinking water; instead of sweet desserts, they begin eating fruit for dessert; instead of sweets, they significantly reduce their consumption by savoring smaller portions less frequently. More vegetables, salads, and fruit are consumed. Then, an amazing thing happens. They begin to actually crave veggies, salads, and fruits! I've seen this in my own life and in countless clients' lives. It gives me confidence to say change what you eat, and you'll change what you crave.

Dig Deeper

Reflection and action:

1. Are you in need of a taste bud rehab? Consider a 30-day break from your sweet habit.

Resources and reading:

1. The Human Microbiome Project of the National Institutes of Health (NIH) - https://commonfund.nih.gov/hmp/

TIP 21 - SET SMARTER GOALS
AND STAY MOTIVATED

"A goal without a plan is just a wish."

Antoine de Saint-Exupéry, French writer

"People often say that motivation doesn't last. Well, neither does bathing – that's why we recommend it daily."

Zig Ziglar, motivational speaker and author

Have you ever made a New Year's resolution to eat healthier or exercise more? If so, you aren't alone. These are the top two New Year's resolutions. While these might sound like noble goals, there's a problem. Without a specific plan to achieve these goals, they most likely will not be achieved.

It's important to set goals. Goals serve as the basis for my work with clients. They give us something to work toward. While I interview clients and have an idea of areas for improvement, it is up to each person to decide what they want to work on first, second, third, etc. Tackling all of their desired and recommended changes at one time is overwhelming. So, we break things down into manageable steps for change. Small changes really do bring big results. One step at a time.

How can we adjust those top New Year's resolutions to better ensure success? We make them SMARTER, a popular acronym used to help make goals more achievable.

SMARTER means the goal is:

- Specific – Clearly define your goal. What food would you like to add? What beverage would you like to decrease? What activity would you like to add?

- Measurable – How much or how often will you eat a food, or how long will you walk, or how many meals or how many days? How will you measure your progress?

- Attainable or achievable – It's important that your goal is attainable. This is why it's important to set your goals individually. What is achievable for each of us may be different. Are you capable of following through?

- Realistic – Remember, progress or improvement is more important than perfection. If you are not a runner, it may be unrealistic to make your goal running a marathon in 30 days. That's extreme, but make sure your goal is realistic for you. It may be walking 15 minutes on Tuesday, Thursday, and Saturday for two weeks and then increase by 5 minutes each week for the rest of the month.

- Time-connected – How often will you do this, or how long will you work on this before reevaluating?

- Evaluate – Is this goal working for you? If you set a goal to exercise at 6 a.m., but you are not a morning person, and rarely wake up in time, then that goal didn't work for you, and you will want to reset the goal to exercise at an alternative time.

- Reward – This can be anything that is a reward for you. For example, if you stop spending money on ice cream, perhaps you will choose to put that money in a jar, and at the end of the 30 or 60 days, you will choose to purchase a massage or piece of jewelry or take a special day trip.

Let's adjust those popular New Year's resolutions. Instead of making a resolution to eat healthier, a SMARTER goal would be:

- I will include at least 1 cup of a green leafy salad or at least a 1/2 cup cooked vegetables with dinner for 5 days a week for the next month.

Instead of making a resolution to exercise more, a SMARTER goal would be:

- I will walk on Tuesday, Saturday, and Sunday for 30 minutes per day for the next month.

Some other ideas for SMARTER goals include:

- I will include foods that contain protein, such as nuts, hummus, or Greek yogurt, as snacks for the next month.

- I will eat fruit at least twice a day for the next 2 months.

To stay motivated, consider what Sir Edmund Hillary, the New Zealand mountaineer and explorer said, "I think it all comes down to motivation. If you really want to do something, you will work hard for it."

Eating for health has similarities to investing in the stock market. How so? With both, it's important to keep your eyes focused on the overall trends and not on the day-to-day changes. It's been said that "the trend is your friend." If you're trying to lose weight, keep your eyes on the big picture and don't get discouraged by a pound or two gained or by a plateau. Remember where you started, keep your eyes on your goal, and keep making healthy choices every day.

Keep in mind that healthy eating habits have many health benefits. Don't make weight loss your only goal. Some other worthwhile benefits include feeling good, having more energy, sleeping well, lowering blood sugar, blood cholesterol, or blood pressure, decreasing heart disease and cancer risk, and supporting a healthy immune system. These are the wonderful benefits of healthy eating and great goals!

As the R in SMARTER reminds us, it's motivating to reward yourself. Put the money you would normally spend on soda, candy, or fast food into a jar to be spent on a special reward of your choice, such as a new outfit, spa treatment, or special trip. Rewarding positive choices and not just weight loss helps you keep your eyes on the benefits of daily healthy choices.

Another way I've personally found that helps me maintain motivation is to stay physically active. Whenever I exercise regularly, no matter what the exercise is, I am more motivated to eat well. I've noticed the same thing with others. People who exercise regularly are more motivated to eat healthy every day and are also motivated to stick with healthy eating habits.

Dig Deeper

Reflection and action:

1. Write a goal to work on this week, using the SMARTER format. For example, do you have a specific food you would like to add, decrease, or eliminate?

2. What keeps you motivated? How could you reward yourself for meeting goals?

Resources and reading:

1. Krieger, E. & James-Enger, K. (2013). *Small changes, big results. Revised and updated.* Clarkson Potter.

TIP 22 - PORTION SIZE MATTERS

"The sharing of food is the basis of social life."

Laurie Colwin, writer and food columnist

The other day, a client told me, "I know what I need to do. I'm just not doing it. The other night, I had Chinese food. I ate a normal serving and I felt full, but I just kept right on eating anyway. I mean, I know what to do. I know I should have stopped, but I didn't. I just kept right on eating even though I was full. I've got to stop that."

Can you relate? At some point in our lives, we probably all can relate. Personally, I overate as a way of life, until my early twenties, when I began to study nutrition, hunger, and fullness. At home, I was often referred to as the "bottomless pit," or even the "human garbage disposal." Not very complimentary, but my love for food was great and I kept eating, despite feeling full. I ate until stuffed and thought that was normal.

Over the years, I have learned many ways to enjoy the foods I love without overeating to the point of feeling stuffed. One of these ways is to share food with others, especially when eating out. When I'm eating out with friends and family who share the same tastes in food, it's great! We may share appetizers, salads, and entrees. This gives us an opportunity to taste more options and even leave room to share dessert.

As registered dietitian nutritionists (RDN), we often say that "all foods can fit" into a healthy menu. This way of thinking baffles many. It even may anger some folks who see nutrition in more black and white terms—the "eat this not that" thinkers. But, sharing food, especially calorie-dense food, significantly decreases calorie intake and allows you to enjoy more options without feeling deprived. Remember, research shows that the first few bites of food are the most satisfying. Dr. Wendy Bazilian, promotes a 3-bite rule, consisting of "ooh, yum, done!"

As I mentioned before, I love fried food. But it doesn't always love me back. Eating fried food can leave me feeling bloated, with indigestion, and promotes weight gain. Even so, vegetable tempura and onion rings, are some of my favorite foods. A serving has about 400-600 calories. A daily or even weekly diet of these items would not only lead to weight gain and indigestion, but these high calorie choices would fill me up and take the place of other healthier nutrient-dense food. My solution? I share an order with family or friends. With eating only one-quarter of the order, I am down to eating about 100-150 calories. This is a significant difference. This leaves me feeling happy and satisfied, instead of deprived and discouraged. It's a win-win.

With "all foods can fit" thinking, the most important things to remember are how often you eat the food, and how much of the food you eat. Portion size matters.

Some examples of foods to eat in shared or "few bites" portions include:

- fried foods
- chips
- ice cream
- cakes, cookies, pies
- candy

Here's some math on the power of sharing portions of "few bites" foods:

1. Small order of French fries: one-half order = 105 calories, 5 grams fat, 13 grams carbohydrates

2. Cheesecake: 1 oz or ¼ cup = 90 calories, 6 grams fat, 8 grams carbohydrates

3. Ice cream: ¼ cup = 65 calories, 3.5 grams fat, 8 grams carbohydrates

4. Chocolate, dark: 1 oz = 150 calories, 8-10 grams fat, 13 grams carbohydrates

5. Hershey kisses, each = 25 calories, 1.5 grams fat, 3 grams carbohydrates

6. Dove chocolate miniatures, each = 30 calories, 2 grams fat, 3 grams carbohydrates

Sharing food and learning to stop by saying "I'm full," saves calories, money, and time because you have leftovers to eat another time, and you will be cooking less. Eating less means spending less. And you don't have to keep buying new clothes because you outgrow the ones you have. That saves money too.

Portions and Serving Sizes

For better health and weight control, serving size matters. Even if you eat healthy food all day long, you may still gain unwanted weight if you don't pay attention to how much you're consuming. Too many people fall into the trap of portion distortion – accepting extra-large portions as normal.

Standard portions have increased over the years. But what's surprising, is just how much they've increased and how many more calories are being consumed today because of it. For example, in 1916 a standard bottle of Coke was 6.5 ounces and 78 calories compared with today's serving of 20 ounces and 240 calories.

To see how much portion sizes have increased, the National Heart Lung and Blood Institute (NHLBI) has a portion distortion quiz at their website. According to the NHLBI, a "portion" is how much food you choose to eat at one time. A "serving" size is the amount of food listed on a product's Nutrition Facts label. The U.S. Food and Drug Administration (FDA) Nutrition Facts information is printed on most packaged foods and tells you the number of calories, fat, carbohydrates, sodium, and other nutrients that are in one serving. Most packaged foods contain more than a single serving in a package.

To help you control how much you eat, it helps to visualize serving sizes. Use the following guidelines. Since we all have different size hands, think of a medium sized hand when using the hand as a guide.

- one cup of cereal is about the size of a baseball or a fist

- 1/2 cup of cooked rice, pasta, fruit, or cooked vegetables is about the size of ½ of a baseball or ½ of a fist

- one medium piece of fruit is the size of a baseball or a fist

- 1 ½ ounces of cheese is about the size of 4 stacked dice

- three ounces of meat is about the size of a deck of cards or a palm

- 2 tablespoons of peanut butter or salad dressing is about the size of a ping pong ball

- 1 tablespoon is about the size of the tip of a thumb

- 1 teaspoon of butter, margarine, or oil is about the size of one pat, one die, or the tip of a finger

Choosing smaller servings or sharing ordinary servings, especially of high fat and high sugar foods, makes a major difference in your overall calorie intake. Consider these calorie comparisons:

- small French fries = 225 calories versus large French fries = 515 calories

- regular cheeseburger = 330 calories versus a quarter pound cheeseburger = 515 calories

- 12 oz. Coke (child's size) = 115 calories versus 32 oz. Coke (large) = 310 calories

Remember, common portions may be equal to 2-3 serving sizes.

Keep a food diary and use measuring spoons and cups to help assess your intake. Visit an RDN for a thorough nutrition evaluation of your usual intake.

If you would like to lose weight, try downsizing your glasses, mugs, plates, or bowls. Research by Dr. Brian Wansink at Cornell Food and Brand Lab showed that by using tall skinny glasses, and eating off smaller plates and bowls, people were satisfied with less, and didn't even notice the difference in intake. How's that for eating skills? As Dr. Wansink says, "Skill power, not willpower."

Some Foods Provide Nutrients but Portions Matter

Some foods are rich in nutrients, but are higher in calories, so if weight control is your goal, they need to be eaten in smaller portions or they may lead to unwanted weight gain. If you are underweight and want to gain weight, these are some foods to add. But if you want to maintain or lose weight, remember, while these foods have many nutritional benefits, portion size still matters. Some of these include:

- nuts
- seeds
- oils, such as extra-virgin olive oil
- avocados
- cheese

Also included in this category is chocolate. Did you know that the most craved food is chocolate? In recent years, research has identified various health benefits of chocolate, especially dark chocolate, including:

- antioxidants that help prevent cholesterol from sticking to artery walls, reducing your risk of a heart attack or stroke

- flavonoids, a type of antioxidant which are the same beneficial compounds found in red wine and tea
    - Of chocolate products, cocoa powder ranks the

highest in flavonoids, followed by dark chocolate and then milk chocolate. Look for dark chocolate with at least 70% cacao for the most health benefits.

- limited amounts of caffeine
  - An average serving of chocolate contains about 5 -10 mg of caffeine, while one cup of coffee contains about 100 -150 mg.

So, while dark chocolate in moderation may be satisfying, remember moderation is key. The next time you feel the stress building, get moving for some health-inducing relief. And refer to the tips in the third section for practical, healthy ways to reduce feeling overwhelmed or stressed.

Dig Deeper

Reflection and action:

1. Use measuring cups to find out how much your glasses, mugs, plates, and bowls hold.

2. This week, try using measuring cups and spoons to help you visualize how much you usually eat and how that compares to serving sizes.

Resources and reading:

1. Wansink, B. (2014). *Slim by design: Mindless eating solutions for everyday life.* William Morrow.

2. National Institutes of Health's Portion Distortion Quiz - https://www.nhlbi.nih.gov/health/educational/wecan/eat-right/portion-distortion.htm

3. Young, L. (2019). *Finally full, finally slim: 30 days to permanent weight loss one portion at a time.* Center Street.

TIP 23 - EAT FOODS THAT
HELP YOU FEEL FULL

"What if you could eat more food, instead of less?"

Barbara Rolls, PhD, nutrition professor, researcher, and author

A re you eating more mindfully? Are you paying better attention to your hunger and your fullness? If so, I hope you've noticed that some foods help you feel your fullness better than others.

Nutrient rich foods that provide more nutrients without being high in calories, are the best choices for helping you to feel your fullness. Foods that provides protein, fiber, and water promote fullness. The same food also helps to prevent or treat some chronic diseases such as type 2 diabetes, high blood cholesterol levels, and certain types of cancer.

Let's look at some foods that helps you to feel full:

- Dairy products are rich in protein and potassium, and milk is also rich in water. Research shows that dairy products help with weight control, blood pressure and blood sugar control.

- Dairy alternatives, soy and pea protein milks, are also rich in protein, potassium, and water.

- Fruits are high in water and fiber. Watermelon is a whopping 92% water.

- Vegetables contain protein, water, and fiber. Fill half your plate with healthy vegetables.

- Beans, peas, and lentils are a unique sub-category of vegetables, also called pulses or legumes. They are higher in protein and fiber than other vegetables, as such, they are excellent substitutes for meat, fish, poultry, and eggs.

• Protein-rich foods, such as fish, poultry, lean beef, pork, eggs, cheese, cottage cheese, and nuts are high in protein, the most satiating nutrient. Even small amounts of protein-rich foods with meals and snacks increase the satiety value of the meal or snack, helping you to feel full longer. Nuts and soy are protein sources that also contain fiber.

• Whole grains foods, such as oatmeal, whole wheat or whole rye breads and cereals, barley, quinoa, and brown rice are high in fiber, which adds to feelings of fullness, keeps bowels regular, and lowers blood cholesterol levels.

• Water, although not a food, provides zero calories and is essential for life. More on water in Tip 33.

Remember to include these foods that help you feel full with your meals and snacks.

Dig Deeper
Reflection and action:
1. Write down what you eat in a day. Are you eating foods with protein, water, and fiber with meals and snacks?

2. If not, what could you add or trade to create meals and snacks that help you feel full?

Resources and reading:
1. Rolls, B. & Hermann, M. (2012). *The ultimate volumetrics diet: Smart, simple, science-based strategies for losing weight and keeping it off.* William Morrows Cookbooks.

2. Seale, S.A., Sherard, T., & Fleming, D. (2010). *The full plate diet.* Bard Press.

TIP 24 - THE POWER OF 100 CALORIES

"We must not, in trying to think about how we can make
a big difference, ignore the small daily differences we
can make which, over time, add up to big differences
that we often cannot foresee."

Marian Wright Edelman, activist

Have you seen the ads on TV claiming to help you lose 14 pounds in one week? This amazing weight loss program may be endorsed by a celebrity. While scrolling on your favorite social media, have you seen a friend's post of a "before and after" photo showing a large amount of weight lost by following the latest weight loss program? These ads are attention grabbing, especially, if you want to lose weight. Unfortunately, weight quickly lost is often weight regained. Research continues to emerge on the topic of why many diets don't work and how small changes can lead to big results.

If you think a small decrease of 100 calories can't make much of a difference, think again. Eating just 100 calories more than you need each day can result in a 10-pound weight gain in a year. Conversely, eating just 100 calories less per day can result in a 10-pound weight loss in a year. Burning just 100 additional calories per day can result in 10 pounds of weight loss in a year. So, if you want to double that, cut 100 calories and add exercise that burns 100 calories to every day. That may result in 20 pounds lost in a year.

What it takes to make this difference can be quite surprising. In looking at 100 calories per day, adding just one tablespoon of oil for cooking adds about 100 calories more than adding just a teaspoon of oil. The difference seems very small, but daily, it is significant.

Here are some examples that are approximately 100 calories:

- 2 teaspoons butter
- 4 Hershey kisses
- ¼ cup premium ice cream
- 12-oz lite beer
- 5 ounces of wine
- 2 chicken nuggets
- 10 potato chips
- 2 slices of bacon

Simple swaps to save approximately 100 calories:

- Drink skim or 1% milk instead of whole.
- Choose baked chicken breast instead of fried chicken breast.
- Use 1 teaspoon oil instead of 1 tablespoon to coat veggies for roasting.
- Use cooking spray instead of butter or oil for sautéing.
- Eat bran or corn flakes instead of sugar-frosted flakes.
- Eat an orange instead of drinking 12 ounces of juice.
- Substitute half of the oil in a baked goods recipe with applesauce.
- Substitute a small size candy to satisfy your sweet tooth instead of a standard size.

Simple activities to burn about 100 calories:

- 30-minute walk at 2 miles per hour
- 10 minutes of aerobic dancing
- 30-minute bike ride at 5 miles per hour
- 10-minute jog at 6 miles per hour
- 30 minutes of light housecleaning
- 15 minutes of scrubbing the floors
- 15 minutes of swimming
- 15-30 minutes of gardening

Dig Deeper

Reflection and action:

1. If you are wanting to lose weight, how could you decrease your intake by 100 calories?

2. How could you burn an extra 100 calories?

3. Pay attention to the minor changes you could be making every day that could lead to big results.

Resources and reading:

1. Krieger, E. & James-Enger, K. (2013). *Small changes, big results. Revised and updated.* Clarkson Potter.

TIP 25 - MAKE PEACE WITH YOUR PLATE

"Call a truce – stop the food fight."

Evelyn Tribole and Elyse Resch, RDNs and authors

W hat comes to mind when you think about a food fight? A cafeteria scene in a movie or family table where folks are slinging food at one another? One of my favorite movies, *It Takes Two*, has an epic food fight scene. But that's not the kind of food fight I'm talking about here. I'm talking about the fight that goes on between your mind, stomach, fork, and plate.

"Eat this, don't eat that," might seem like good advice. Many clients tell me, "Just tell me what to eat." People think that is the easier way. But after three decades of nutrition counseling, I know that people don't change because of information, they change because of transformation, which is an inside-out job, not an outside-in job.

Internal stimulation, such as listening to your body's cues for hunger and fullness and listening to your body for cues about which foods and how much of those foods to eat, help you to feel your best. These are the best ways to transform your eating habits. External stimulation, such as a parent telling you to eat all your vegetables before you can have dessert, or to clean your plate because children are starving in other parts of the world, is not an effective way to motivate change. Instead, this causes a war, not only between you and your parents, but also between you and the food on your plate.

Quit the Clean Plate Club

Did you grow up being taught the virtues of being a member of the "clean plate club?" I did and so did many of my clients.

Some people were given the reward of dessert or even stickers on a chart for cleaning their plates. Most of the people in my generation—baby boomers—were taught that we needed to eat everything on our plates, because "There are starving children in the world." While I totally support helping to feed children all over the world, it's time to realize that eating everything on your plate doesn't help feed starving children anywhere and it may add unwanted calories and pounds.

This is especially important as we look at decreasing food waste. I've heard the same advice about cleaning your plate in reference to decreasing food waste. There are better ways to decrease food waste, and they will be discussed in the next tip.

Last Supper Thinking

Did you ever know someone, or maybe even yourself, who binged the night before starting their next new diet? This "last supper" thinking can happen repeatedly and fosters a most unhealthy relationship with your plate and weight gain.

Black and White Thinking

This type of extreme thinking can be harmful. For example, black and white thinking could be "I'm either on a diet or I'm not." If I'm on a diet, I'm following a set of rigid food rules. If I'm not on a diet, then I am splurging on anything and everything that I want. These two extremes are both unhealthy. Healthy eating habits are best when you can live with them forever.

Diets Don't Work

One of the many reasons that diets don't work is because health is an inside job and not an outside job. Diets are equated with deprivation. Deprivation is psychologically a catalyst for overindulging. Overindulging or bingeing leads to guilt and shame and the cycle goes on and on. Instead of the deprive, binge, guilt, shame cycle, resolve to make peace with your plate and to listen to your own body. Listen to your gut about what foods you enjoy, what foods help you to feel good, how much food helps you to feel satisfied and not stuffed, and you will make peace with your plate and stop the food fight.

Dig Deeper

Reflection and action:

1. Examine your thoughts and feelings about food. Do you have any distorted thinking or "stinking thinking?" Do you need to make peace with your plate?

2. Commit to working on having a healthy relationship with the food on your plate. What could you change to help you make peace with your plate?

Resources and reading:

1. Tribole, E. & Resch, E. (2012). *Intuitive eating.* St. Martin's Griffin.

2. Wansink, B. (2011). *Mindless eating: Why we eat more than we think.* Hay House.

TIP 26 - THE IMPORTANCE OF A PLAN AND TIPS TO REDUCE FOOD WASTE

"If you fail to plan, you are planning to fail."
Benjamin Franklin

<u>*Food*</u>
1. Buy it with thought.
2. Cook it with care.
3. Serve just enough.
4. Save what will keep.
5. Eat what would spoil.
6. Home grown is best.
7. Don't waste it.

1917 U.S. Food Administration

D o you think it is quick and easy to stop at the drive-through on your way home? Think again. How many times do you wait in line? Special order? And what about the mistakes? It can be stressful and frustrating, especially when you're super hungry. Then, fast food isn't so fast after all. And that bag of fries, are they half eaten before you even get home?

Statistics show that if you don't have a plan for dinner, you will more likely go out to eat. The goal is to make it quicker, tastier, and easier to prepare meals at home than to stop at a drive through. For some, this will mean writing up weekly menus. For others, it means keeping a well-stocked pantry, fridge, and freezer. For some, it can be a combo of the two. There is power in a well-stocked kitchen: counters, refrigerator, freezer, and pantry!

Keeping your kitchen well-stocked better ensures you have all the components needed for a healthy meal. Here is a sample list of items (not exhaustive) to keep handy for quick meals. Stock what you like. No one list fits all. There's no sense in having foods you won't eat.

Kitchen counter:
- fresh fruit and vegetables best kept at room temperature, such as bananas, peaches, avocados, and tomatoes

Pantry and cupboards:
- whole grains, such as pasta and quinoa
- rice (brown, wild rice, red, jasmine, or basmati)
- dried herbs and spices
- canned fruit in water or its own juice
- canned vegetables – no added salt or low sodium
- beans, such as cannellini, kidney, garbanzo and black (canned or dried)
- broths – low sodium vegetable, beef, and chicken
- onions
- potatoes
- soups – low sodium
- dried fruits
- canned or pouches of protein foods, such as tuna, chicken, salmon, and sardines

Freezer:
- vegetables, plain and mixes, such as mixed vegetables for soups or vegetable blends for stews
- fruits with no added sugar
- fish, poultry, and meats
- vegetarian items, such as edamame, vegetarian crumbles, or sausage substitutes
- frozen meals – limit to 600-700 mg sodium per serving

Refrigerator:
- dairy or dairy substitute of choice – milk or specialized milk that are easier to digest for some such as A2 or

Lactaid, soy, almond, oat, or other milk substitutes of your choice; cream, half and half, or nondairy options
- cheese – cow, sheep, goat, or nondairy
- yogurt – dairy, or substitute such as soy or coconut milk
- fruit – apples, oranges, grapefruits, lemons, limes, mandarin oranges, grapes, and fruit in season or of your choice
- vegetables – lettuces, leafy greens, peppers, carrots, celery, cucumbers, mushrooms, and veggies in season or of your choice
- eggs
- butter or olive oil spread
- pickled vegetables
- salsa, hummus, or guacamole
- ketchup, mustard, mayonnaise, and other condiments of your choice

Tips to reduce food waste from your pantry, fridge, and freezer:
- Check your own inventory before heading to the store. Use food you saved-over at least once weekly to keep your inventory fresh.
- Move older food products to the front of the pantry, fridge, or freezer. This ensures that you use up older items first.
- Substitute items in recipes with what you already have on hand, when possible. For example, if a recipe calls for kale, but you have spinach, use the spinach instead. Or if a recipe calls for black beans, but you have white beans, consider using the white beans.
- Routinely eat out of your freezer weekly or monthly. Otherwise, it's easy to forget what is in the freezer. Consider keeping a list of items on the door, too.

Some ways to use more of your produce:
- Use the tops of root vegetables like turnips, carrots, and

radishes. These can be used the same as other greens. Try chopping them into salads or sauteing them with garlic and olive oil. I like to mix them in with other more familiar greens, such as spinach or baby kale.

- If not used in your recipe, save stalks of broccoli and cauliflower, and store these in the freezer to use when making a creamy or cheesy soup.

Dig Deeper

Reflection and action:

1. Check out your kitchen. Where are you storing food? If you're storing foods on your counters, make changes to store most foods out of sight, except fruit and vegetables, which has been shown to help with weight control.

2. Check your pantry, refrigerator, and freezer. Are you well-stocked? If not, consider stocking up, so you are able to put together a well-balanced meal in minutes.

3. Take stock of how much food is wasted in your home and work towards decreasing your household food waste.

Resources and reading:

1. Krieger, E. (2009). *So easy.* John Wiley and Sons.

2. Krieger, E. (2019). *Whole in one.* Da Capo Lifelong Books.

3. Geagan, K. (2009). *Go green get lean.* Rodale.

4. Rust, R. (2022). *Zero waste cooking for dummies.* For Dummies.

TIP 27 - QUICK AND EASY MEALS

"One can say everything best over a meal."

George Eliot, English writer

People often ask me for meal plans. I bought a few different meal planning computer programs and used them professionally, even though I never really got into using them personally. People are often surprised by this. However, if you know the components of a healthy meal, it simplifies meal planning, and you aren't bound by food ideas that someone else is offering you.

Knowing the components that make up a healthy meal, as reviewed extensively in Tip 4, is the key to menu planning. The website, ChooseMyPlate.com thoroughly discusses the basics of meal planning using the MyPlate icon/graphic as the tool. There are also a couple of weeks of menu ideas for people on a budget included on the website.

In summary, using the plate planner for adults, fill half of your plate with vegetables or vegetables and fruits, one-quarter of the plate with protein, and one-quarter of your plate with whole grain or starchy foods. Fruit is included 3 times per day with meals or snacks. Dairy products or dairy substitutes are included 2-3 times per day. It's really that simple.

But since so many people ask me for dinner ideas, I designed a brochure that offered suggestions. Keep in mind that you don't have to cook a full meal every night. Leftovers, or saved-overs, as I write about in the next couple of tips, allow you to cook less. It's good to have at least 5-10 quick and easy meals that you are completely comfortable preparing. While I love to experiment with new recipes, I have my "go-to" favorite meals, too. The following suggestions include the components discussed on the MyPlate icon.

#1 -Spinach and Stars Soup (recipe included below)
Whole grain crackers or rolls
Tossed salad
Strawberries or seasonal fruit

#2 -Baked Chicken with roasted sweet potatoes, turnips & carrots
Blueberries or seasonal fruit

#3 -Spaghetti with meat or marinara sauce with vegetables, such as mushrooms
Parmesan cheese
Tossed salad or Caesar salad with or without anchovies
Sliced oranges or seasonal fruit

#4 -Stir-Fry: beef, pork, chicken, or shrimp
Stir-fried vegetables, such as snow peas, carrots, mushrooms, or onions
Brown rice
Peaches, apricots, or seasonal fruit

#5 -Barbecue or oven roasted herb chicken
Quinoa or baked potato
Glazed carrots
Kiwi or seasonal fruit

* * *

Spinach and Stars Soup

6 cups chicken stock (homemade or low sodium box)
3/4-1 cup star shaped pastina (depending on thickness desired)
1 pound of fresh spinach or 1 (10 oz) package frozen chopped spinach, thawed and drained
1 egg
1/4 cup grated Parmesan cheese
1/8 teaspoon pepper

Heat chicken broth to boiling. Add pastina stars and simmer about 5 minutes. Chop and add spinach or cook frozen spinach in microwave, according to package directions and drain all excess liquid. Add fresh or drained spinach to soup. Crack egg into small bowl and mix well. Add egg to soup, drizzling in small drops at a time. Add cheese and pepper and stir. Serves 6.

❋ ❋ ❋

Breakfast ideas include oatmeal or whole grain cereals with fruit and nuts, milk or milk substitutes, such as soy milk. You'll also find a wonderful vegetable cheese omelet with whole grain toast and fruit, as well as Greek yogurt with fruit, nuts and avocado topped whole grain toast.

Lunch ideas include vegetable soup with turkey or a peanut butter sandwich with fruit. Bean soup with tossed salad and fruit, and tuna on top of a tossed salad with whole grain crackers and piece of fruit are some delightful additional lunch suggestions. Snack ideas include hummus and raw vegetables, yogurt and fruit, nut butters with crackers, or nuts and fruit.

As you can see, meal planning is as simple as including your favorite protein foods, vegetables, starches or whole grains, and fruits. Dairy foods can also be included with meals or snacks.

Dig Deeper

Reflection and action:

1. What are some of your favorite meals?

2. Write down 5 meals that can be your go-to, easy balanced meals.

Resources and reading:

1. Andrews, L. C. (2021). *Heart healthy meal prep: 6 weekly plans for low-sodium, high-flavor, grab-and-go meals.* Rockridge Press.

2. Nicholson, S. (2010). *7-Day menu planner for dummies.* For Dummies.

3. USDA MyPlate Recipes with videos and more - https://www.myplate.gov/myplate-kitchen/recipes

TIP 28 - RETHINKING LEFTOVERS

"Cutting food waste is a delicious way of saving money,
helping to feed the world and protect the planet."

Tristram Stuart, author

According to the United States Department of Agriculture (USDA), about 40% of our food supply is wasted, with the average American family of four throwing out $1,500 in food per year. We can all make changes to improve this problem. Mindful shopping and mindful eating habits encourage us to intentionally choose, prepare, eat, and store foods.

Makeovers are in demand these days. I saw an ad for a plastic surgeon that promised, "The new and improved YOU!" I think it's about time we give leftovers a makeover as well!

The name leftovers sound so stale. It conjures up images of old food, left in the refrigerator for who knows how long? But it doesn't have to be that way. For example, meal prep is about intentionally cooking one day and then preparing the leftovers for future meals. Prepare once and eat more than once. That's what meal prep is about.

I was raised eating leftovers. I enjoyed them for breakfast, lunch, dinner, or snacks. They didn't last longer than one or two meals, so I didn't really get tired of eating the same thing too many times in a row. Meals like spaghetti, lasagna, chili, vegetable soup, or a Filipino favorite, adobo, all seem to get better with time. The flavors improve and quality doesn't suffer.

Sometimes, the same people who stock their freezers with frozen entrees and snacks, turn their noses up at leftovers. But isn't it similar, and maybe better, to make your own homemade frozen meals from your fresh foods, and your recipes? Instead of calling these leftovers, let's call our foods eaten for more than one meal: *saved-overs.*

Saved-overs implies a mindful, intentional purpose in saving foods for later. When cooking, it makes sense to cook extra to save for later. Here's what you're saving:

- Time – You only make the meal once and then you enjoy it multiple times. For people with limited time due to busy schedules, this is time you have for doing other things.

- Energy – It takes energy, yours and electricity or gas, to make food, so why not make enough to save over for another meal?

- Money – By saving your food to eat in the next day or two, or to freeze for later use, you get more food for your dollar. Keep a marker nearby to date your frozen food.

If you stretch your food dollars, you'll be less likely to stretch your waistline. Eating less at the present meal saves calories. Most people can benefit from this. Learning to be satisfied with less and saving food for another meal will help you not overeat, which will help prevent unwanted weight gain.

When possible, try to store food in clear containers. One problem with saving food in the refrigerator for another meal is that it often gets buried—we forget about them until we clean the fridge. We've all experienced the long-forgotten leftovers that look more like a science experiment than food. YUCK!

But the problem isn't with saving the food, or the leftovers or saved-overs themselves. The problem is that we forget they are there. The solution: Store food in clear containers or freezer bags so that you can always SEE what you have.

If you can't see it, you forget about it. That's happened to me many times before my switch to clear containers. You can also keep a white board nearby to write what foods are inside the fridge, so that everyone in the house can quickly see available choices.

According to the Food Safety and Inspection Service (FSIS) of USDA, most saved-over foods can be kept in the refrigerator for 3-4 days or frozen for 3-4 months. Although safe indefinitely, frozen foods can lose moisture and flavor when stored for longer times in the freezer.

Dig Deeper

Reflection and action:

1. Evaluate the contents of your pantry, refrigerator, and freezer and plan to build your menus using those items.

2. If you don't already have clear containers or freezer bags, buy some.

TIP 29 - GIVE SAVED-OVERS A TASTE-OVER

"At the end of the week, my husband and I do a leftovers dinner, where we have to use whatever's in the fridge. It's sort of a game."

Lake Bell, actor, screenwriter, and director

Many clients tell me that they don't like to eat the same foods two days in a row. Consider giving your saved-over foods a taste-over. A taste-over is the same food prepared in a different way so that it tastes new. Your family may not even realize it. But if they do and they still don't like the idea, then I recommend freezing foods immediately after cooking to use in a taste-over in a week or more later. As mentioned in the previous tip, most frozen prepared foods maintain excellent quality for 3-4 months.

The most common taste-overs occur after cooking the enormous Thanksgiving Day turkey. When you roast any poultry, including turkey or chicken, it makes a wonderful meal that day. But it also makes multiple optional meals for later. Use it over the next few days or freeze it in meal size portions to be used in casseroles and soups later. Once in the freezer, the key is not forgetting that it is there. I recommend including your frozen foods in your menus, to ensure using up the delicious, homemade frozen foods. Keeping a list on the freezer door is a good reminder. Planning to routinely check the freezer and eat from the freezer is also a good habit. Here are some examples of taste-overs:

Roast chicken or turkey:
- chicken noodle soup or any other kind of soup (e.g., white chicken chili, chicken corn)

- casseroles, such as chicken/turkey broccoli casserole (e.g., chicken divan)
- chicken salad for sandwiches or salads
- chicken pot pie
- chicken and gravy over waffles or mashed potatoes or mashed cauliflower
- buffalo chicken dip

Roast beef:
- beef salad
- beef vegetable soup or other soups
- hot roast beef over whole grain bread or mashed potatoes
- stir-fries, such as beef with broccoli over stir-fried rice or riced cauliflower
- beef and cheese omelet

Mashed potatoes:
- potato pancakes
- pierogies
- gnocchi

Think about enhancing your leftovers or taste-overs with spices. They add delicious flavor, and many have anti-inflammatory properties. These include:
- turmeric, curry powder, ginger. garlic, chili peppers, basil, cinnamon, rosemary, and thyme, as desired
  ○ Turmeric and ginger are powerful, natural anti-inflammatory agents.

Add international flavor to stir fries with small variations, such as:
- Indian – use basmati rice, spinach, onions, tomatoes, curry powder, almonds, and milk
- Italian – use basil, oregano, rosemary, parsley, olive oil, and top with Parmesan cheese
- Japanese – use soba or udon noodles, bok choy, shitake

mushrooms and peppers, fresh ginger, sesame oil, soy sauce, and top with sesame seeds

- Thai – use jasmine rice, cabbage, celery, carrots, sesame oil, Thai chili paste, fish sauce, lime juice, and top with peanuts

Remember, eating saved-overs is a great way to fight food waste. Other ways are included in the next tip.

Dig Deeper

Reflection and action:

1. What are your favorite ways to use saved-overs?

2. Experiment with various herbs and spices to give a taste-over to your saved-overs this week.

Resources and reading:

1. Patel, G. (2011). *Blending science with spices.* Feeding Health.

2. Amidor, T. (2017). *The healthy meal prep cookbook.* Rockridge Press.

3. The James Beard Foundation. (2018). Waste *not: How to get the most from your food.* Rizzoli.

4. Excellent resource with practical tools to help families decrease food waste from the United States Environmental Protection Agency. https://www.epa.gov/sustainable-management-food/food-too-good-waste-implementation-guide-and-toolkit#docs

TIP 30 - EAT LOCAL AND GROW A GARDEN

"To plant a garden is to believe in tomorrow."

Audrey Hepburn, actor and humanitarian

There's nothing like a fresh tomato from the garden! Tomato lovers wait with anticipation all year to savor that special summer flavor. When I was growing up, I didn't like fresh tomatoes. Looking back, I can hardly believe it! One of my closest friend's family grew tomatoes every summer, and she tried in vain to turn me into a fresh-from-the-vine tomato convert. But the powerful experience of eating something that didn't taste good overwhelmed my adventurous spirit. As a nutrition educator, I remember this and recommend seasonal produce when cooking for others that may be trying something for the first time. A negative taste experience can stay with someone for years.

The word locavore is used to describe those who eat a diet consisting of local food. What that "local" area is varies, but it is generally recognized as foods harvested from within an area of a 100-mile radius (locavore was a New Oxford American Dictionary's word of the year in 2005). Now, I love promoting fresh, locally grown food, including tomatoes. Going to the farmers' market evokes excitement in me similar to a trip to Disney World. It's one of my happy places.

There are so many reasons why eating local food is so exciting and important. Here are some of my favorites:

- save money – fresh, seasonal foods are less expensive
- save energy – less gas used to move the food
- support local growers and sustainable farming practices
- be healthy – fresh, seasonal foods are more flavorful

which encourages increased intake of fresh fruits and veggies, healthy vitamins, minerals, and phytonutrients that fight disease and promote health

And even better, how about growing your own garden. It's been said that "Gardening is cheaper than therapy, and you get tomatoes." I know for sure it's therapeutic for me, especially when weeding seems like a form of meditation. Gardening is a fantastic way to get exercise and you can't get more local than your own backyard! But even if you don't plant a garden, you can still enjoy the flavors of nutritious fresh produce.

Some Health Benefits of Gardening

1. Exercise - According to the National Institutes of Health, light gardening burns approximately 330 calories per hour (average based on a 154-pound person). That's only 50 calories less per hour than hiking, the same as dancing and golfing (while walking and carrying clubs) for an hour, and more than bicycling (290 biking less than 10 mph) and walking (3.5 mph) for the same amount of time.

2. Improves mood and helps manage stress, anxiety, and depression – Gardening, like other physical activities, increases our hormones that help us feel good, such as serotonin; and it helps to decrease our stress hormone, cortisol. Also, according to a study in *Neuroscience*, soil contains healthy bacteria that increase serotonin.

3. Improves bone health – Like other weight bearing exercises, gardening helps prevent the risk of developing osteoporosis by helping to keep bones strong.

4. Increases vitamin D – Vitamin D, also known as the sunshine vitamin, is made by our bodies when skin is exposed to sunlight. According to a study reported in *Nutrition Research* in 2011, it

is estimated that over 40% of the U.S. population is deficient in vitamin D. Just 30 minutes of gardening for 3 days per week, is recommended to keep vitamin D levels adequate.

5. Mindfulness and meditation – Digging in dirt is a spiritual experience for me. Planting seeds that will produce delicious, nutritious food is rewarding. It requires concentration and focus. I know most people don't enjoy pulling weeds, and neither do I, but after a while, there is a rhythm that develops, and just being in nature helps us be more aware of our surroundings. I think Dorothy Frances Gurney, an English poet and hymn writer, must have felt it, too, when she penned these lines in her poem, "God's Garden:"

> "The kiss of the sun for pardon
> The song of the birds for mirth,
> One is nearer God's heart in a garden
> Than anywhere else on earth."

Dig Deeper

Reflection and action:

1. Do you go to your local farmers' markets? Write the dates and times that work for you on your calendar, so you will remember.

2. Do you grow a garden? If not, buy a few pots and plant a cherry tomato and some herbs. These are easy to grow and may inspire more gardening.

Resources and reading:

1. For farmers' markets close to your home visit www.localharvest.org. To find a farmers' market in your area visit: https://www.ams.usda.gov/local-food-directories/farmersmarkets.

2. Your Guide to Physical Activity and Your Heart. U.S. Department of Health and Human Services, National Institutes of Health, National Heart, Lung, and Blood Institute 2006 https://

www.nhlbi.nih.gov/files/docs/public/heart/phy_active.pdf

3. Haugan, J. (2016). *The mom's guide to a nourishing garden.* https://jenhaugen.com/book/

4. NPR - https://www.npr.org/sections/ thesalt/2012/02/17/147050691/can-gardening-help-troubled-minds-heal.

5. Forrest K., & Stuhldreher W. (2011). Prevalence and correlates of vitamin D deficiency in US adults. *Nutrition Research*, 31(1), 48-54. https://www.doi.org/10.1016/j.nutres.2010.12.001

TIP 31 - EAT MORE VEGETABLES AND FRUITS

"Fruits and vegetables, the best edibles."
Author Unknown

"We should all be eating fruits and vegetables as if our lives depend on it – because they do."
Michael Greger, physician author, speaker

According to the Centers for Disease Control and Prevention, Americans are not eating enough vegetables and fruits. In fact, only one in ten adults are meeting the federal recommendations for 1.5-2 cups of fruit per day and 2-3 cups of vegetables per day.

When examining the diets of people who live the longest and healthiest lives, we see their diets are high in vegetables and fruits. In looking at research for preventing Alzheimer's and dementia, we again see the benefits of eating a lot of vegetables and fruits. In fact, early in my career, I heard it said that vegetables and fruits are a form of health insurance.

Everyone I interview tells me they like fruit, and although less, most people do like vegetables. Yet, meeting the recommended number of servings per day seems to be the biggest challenge for most of my clients. It's a worthwhile goal, however, as the potential benefits show:

- decreased risk of certain types of cancer
- decreased risk of heart disease
- decreased calorie intake with improved weight control
- improved immunity
- improved vision health
- healthier aging

- improved memory
- improved urinary tract health

Fruits and vegetables are rich in vitamins, minerals, and disease-fighting phytonutrients. These benefits from diets high in vegetables and fruits cannot be achieved simply by taking supplements. That's why it's important to try to get your nutrients from food first. Food is the first line of defense. This is most likely because there are many healthy compounds in vegetables and fruits that have not yet been identified. And most supplements don't contain the important fiber found in eating vegetables and fruit. As my dear friend and registered dietitian nutritionist colleague, Cindy Held says, "Nature's packaging is impossible to mimic in a pill."

Tips to increase fruits and veggies in your diet include:

- Add fresh or frozen berries or bananas to your morning cereal or yogurt.

- Keep dried fruit in your car or desk for a quick snack.

- Mix fresh or frozen fruit with yogurt, milk or plant-based milk alternative, such as soy, almond, or oat milk for a refreshing fruit smoothie.

- Mix ¼ cup of 100% fruit juice with sparkling water for a cool fruit spritzer.

- Keep your pantry and freezer stocked with canned (in juice or water) or frozen (without added sugar) fruit for variety and when out of fresh produce.

- Grow a vegetable garden. There's nothing like a plentiful supply of fresh veggies in season.

- Shop regularly at farmers' markets in your area for flavorful fresh veggies and fruit.

- Try vegetable toppings on your pizza.

- Eat a salad at least once a day.

- Stock your pantry and freezer with canned (without added salt) and frozen (without added sauces or salt) veggies for variety and when out of fresh produce.

- Plan to include fruits and veggies with every meal and snack. Even breakfast can include veggies, such as baby spinach or kale in a smoothie; mushrooms, onions, and peppers in an omelet; or refreshing vegetable juice over ice.

The Produce for Better Health Foundation promotes eating more fruits and vegetables through their "Have a Plant" campaign. Their website, listed below, offers simple ways to add more fruits and veggies to your day. It offers expert advice, nutrition and storage information, shopping tips, healthy menus and recipes, kid-friendly recipes, and healthy tips, as well as ways to save money using fruits and veggies. I highly recommend you check it out for ideas to help you add more vegetables and fruits to your daily meals.

Dig Deeper

Reflection and action:
1. Are you eating at least 1.5-2 cups of fruit per day and 2-3 cups of vegetables per day?

2. Write down a SMARTER goal to help you eat your vegetables and fruits every day. For example, I will eat a vegetable-based salad with lunch or dinner at least 5 days each week. I will eat fruit as a snack at least 5 days a week.

Resources and reading:
1. Produce for Better Health "Have a Plant" campaign - https://fruitsandveggies.org/

2. Palmer, S. (2012). *The plant powered diet.* The Experiment.

TIP 32 - LIMIT SUGAR

"Eat less sugar. You're sweet enough already."

Author Unknown

A high sugar diet is associated with increased cavities, inflammation, higher blood pressure, weight gain, and increased risk for diabetes, fatty liver disease, and heart disease.

The average American consumes an estimated ¼ - ½ pound of sugar each day! That's the equivalent of 30–60 teaspoons of sugar each day. Since each teaspoon of sugar supplies 4 grams of carbohydrate and 16 calories, that adds up to 480—960 calories.

The Dietary Guidelines for Americans (DGA) recommends that adults limit added sugars to less than 10% of total calories. That would be about 10 teaspoons of sugar, 40 grams, or 160 calories for a 1600 calorie diet and 12 teaspoons, 50 grams, or 200 calories for a 2000 calorie diet.

The American Heart Association recommends no more than 9 teaspoons of added sugar per day for men, which equals 36 grams or 150 calories from added sugar and no more than 6 teaspoons of added sugar per day for women, or 24 grams or 100 calories from added sugar. This is the same amount (6 teaspoons) maximum recommended for children.

What are added sugars? Added sugars are sugars and syrups that are added to foods or drinks during processing or preparation. Examples include sucrose, dextrose, corn syrup, honey, syrups, and agave nectar. This doesn't include naturally occurring sugars such as those in fruit, milk, or vegetables. According to the DGAs, people who eat a lot of sugar don't get as many nutrients as people who eat lower-sugar diets. This is because high sugar foods often replace nutrient-rich foods.

According to the DGAs, sugar-sweetened beverages, such as sodas, sports drinks, energy drinks, fruit drinks, and sweetened coffees and teas contribute over 40% of the daily intake of added sugars. It's time to rethink our drinks (Tip 33).

Here are some ways to help you cut down on your sugar intake:

- Think before you drink. Coined "liquid candy" by the Center for Science in the Public Interest, sweet drinks are by far the biggest source of sugar in the average American's diet. Liquid calories add up fast. One 12-ounce can of soda contains about 10 teaspoons of sugar and one 20-ounce bottle contains about 16 teaspoons. And bottled iced teas and energy drinks often contain as much sugar as sodas.

- Read food labels. This can help to identify added sugars. Since 2018, added sugars are required to be on the food label. (No more confusion about whether the sugar is naturally occurring in milk or fruit). Added sugar goes by many names, including sugar, brown sugar, raw sugar, corn sweetener, corn syrup, high-fructose corn syrup, sucrose, glucose, and dextrose.

- Choose nutrient rich foods first. These include fruits and vegetables, lean meat, poultry, fish, eggs, beans, and nuts; whole, fiber-rich grain foods; and milk, cottage cheese, cheese, and yogurt.

- Make snacks count. While some people think snacks are a bad idea, snacks can be important to help us meet our nutrient needs, control hunger, regulate blood sugar levels and mood, and manage weight. Combining a source of protein with a vegetable, fruit, or whole grain helps provide a nourishing, filling snack. Some ideas include: fruit with nuts, such as apple with nut butter, vegetables with hummus, yogurt with fruit, whole grain crackers and cheese or nut butter, and cereal with fruit.

- Pay attention to portions. Choose small servings or share high-calorie, high-sugar desserts when you splurge. Try a child's servings of ice cream, a miniature chocolate, or an extra-small mocha cappuccino. While often not listed on the menu, child size servings, or extra-small sizes, or even a taste are often available if you ask.

- Eat mindfully. When you indulge in sweets, pay attention while you are eating, and savor the flavor of every bite. The first few bites are the most satisfying, so enjoy them immensely, and you will be satisfied with less.

- Drink water. Water is naturally calorie-free and sugar-free. Sparkling water, seltzer water, or carbonated water spritzers are refreshing options. These can be flavored with lemon, lime, or orange wedges, or a splash (a tablespoon) of 100% fruit juice. More tips related to water are in Tip 33.

- Eat fruit. Fruit has been referred to as nature's candy. Naturally sweet, fruit is refreshing, satisfying, and nutritious. Fresh fruit is high in water and fiber, both of which help increase fullness and satisfaction while helping you eat less.

- Limit sweets, such as candy, cookies, cakes, and pies. High in sugar and often high in fat, these foods are calorie-dense, which is the opposite of nutrient-dense or nutrient-rich. Enjoy these foods in moderation, but a steady diet can derail your best efforts for health and wellness.

Dig Deeper

Reflection and action:
1. Are you eating and/or drinking more added sugar than recommended?

2. Set a SMARTER goal for ways to decrease added sugars.

Resources and reading:
1. Harvard Health Publishing. (2019, November 5). *The sweet danger of sugar.* https://www.health.harvard.edu/heart-health/the-sweet-danger-of-sugar

2. Quick tips for reading food labels from the Food and Drug Administration - https://www.fda.gov/media/131162/download

TIP 33 - RETHINK YOUR DRINK: WATER

"I believe that water is the only drink for a wise man."

Henry David Thoreau

Water! There's nothing quite as thirst quenching. Our bodies seem to crave water. And no wonder. More than half our weight comes from water. The body loses about 2-3 quarts of water every day. And if you're exercising or doing physical work in the heat, the loss can be much more.

We need water to:

- help move food through the digestive tract
- carry nutrients and eliminate waste products
- maintain body temperature
- help prevent kidney stones

How much water do we need? Needs vary depending on your weight, age, sex, calorie needs, level of fitness, activity level, health status, and the environmental temperature and humidity.

The Adequate Intake (AI) for total water set by the Dietary Reference Intake Committee of the National Academy Sciences is 125 ounces (about 15 cups) per day for men and 91 ounces (about 11 cups) per day for women. Their report states that about 80% of the estimated total water intake is met by consuming water and beverages, while the other 20% is derived from foods.

For a quick estimate, experts at the Mayo Clinic recommend dividing weight (in pounds) by two to calculate daily water needs (in ounces). For example, to calculate the fluid needs of a 150-pound person's water needs:

150 divided by 2 = 75 ounces per day, then divide
by 8 to convert the amount into cups:
75 divided by 8 = approximately 9.5 cups per day

Recommendations for water may also be called fluid recommen-dations and include fluid from all sources, including beverages and food sources. Many of the foods we eat contain 80-95% water. Caffeine-containing beverages, including some sodas, coffee, tea, and energy drinks have a slight diuretic effect which increases fluid losses if ingested in large quantities.

According to Nancy Clark, author of *Nancy Clark's Sports Nutrition Guidebook*, the simplest way to tell if you are getting enough water is to check the color and quantity of your urine. If your urine is dark and scanty, it is concentrated metabolic wastes and you need to drink more fluids. Urine should be pale yellow. Some vitamin supplements can color the urine, though, so this is not always a reliable indicator.

A very active person may want to check their weight before and after exercise. For every pound lost, they should drink 16 ounces of water to replace fluids lost. Signs of dehydration in-clude thirst, fatigue, headache, weakness, vague discomfort, loss of appetite, dry mouth, reduction in urine, and difficulty con-centrating.

Some tips to help you increase your water intake include:

- Keep a pitcher of water in the refrigerator that contains the amount of water you need daily.

- Keep water with you – on your desk, in your car, on your kitchen counter, or by your favorite chair.

- Spritzers - Flavor water with a slice of lemon or lime. Try seltzer water, club soda or sparkling mineral water flavored with lemon, lime, orange, or a splash of fruit juice.

- Infused waters – Cut or slightly crush fruits, vegetables, and herbs to release flavors. Add to water for at least 4-6 hours or overnight. You don't need a special pitcher or bottle with an infuser, but they are nice. Some great combos include:
lemon, lime, and mint; strawberries, pineapple, and grapes; cucumber, ginger, and mint; oranges, blueberries, and basil; and cucumber, lemon, lime, and basil.

- Eat broth-based soups and water-rich fruits and vegetables. Examples of water-rich vegetables and fruits include cantaloupe, watermelon, strawberries, lettuce, cabbage, celery, spinach, and cooked squash.

Dig Deeper

Reflection and action:

1. How much water do you drink? Measure your glasses and calculate how much you are drinking in a day. Does it meet your needs?

2. If needed, set SMARTER goals to increase water intake.

3. Try making an infused water this week from the ideas above.

Resources and reading:

1. Dietary Reference Intakes - https://ods.od.nih.gov/HealthInformation/Dietary_Reference_Intakes.aspx

2. Clark, N. (2019). *Nancy Clark's Sports Nutrition Guidebook*, Human Kinetics.

TIP 34 - RETHINK YOUR DRINK:
TEA, COFFEE, AND ALCOHOL

"You can't get a cup of tea big enough or a
book long enough to suit me."

C. S. Lewis, British writer

There's nothing like relaxing by a crackling fire and sipping soothing hot tea, especially on a cold damp day. And in the summer, nothing is quite as refreshing as freshly steeped iced tea. Next to water, tea is the most popular beverage in the world.

White, Green, Black, and Oolong Teas

White, green, black, and oolong teas all come from the same plant, Camellia sinensis. How the fresh leaves of the tea plant are processed and their level of contact with oxygen determines the resulting types of tea. Regardless of what kind, I enjoy and drink tea every day—iced or hot. With so many choices on the store shelves, the possibilities are endless.

The benefits of tea are no secret. Tea has ridden a wave of positive reports for many years now. Some benefits include:

- naturally contains no calories

- contains about half of the amount of caffeine as coffee; one cup contains about 50 milligrams of caffeine

- rich in the beneficial polyphenols, including flavanols, theaflavins, and catechins; these act as antioxidants in the body and provide many health benefits

While more studies are needed to confirm these health benefits, it makes sense to include tea as part of a healthy, delicious lifestyle. If you prefer a sweeter tea, try fruit flavored tea such as pomegranate or blueberry green. If you prefer spicy, then try chai, lemon ginger, or cinnamon spice black tea. If you are sensitive to caffeine, or are avoiding it for any reason, decaffeinated and most herbal tea are an option.

Herbal Tea

While herbal teas are called tea in the United States, they are called tisanes in Europe. They are not made from the same Camellia sinensis plant as white, green, and black tea. Instead, these teas are made from dried herbs. Some also have added spices, flowers, fruit, seeds, roots, or leaves of other plants. They do not typically contain caffeine like traditional teas, so they make an excellent choice for those avoiding caffeine. Herbal teas also contain health-promoting polyphenols, but this amount varies, based on the plant sources in the tea.

Coffee

Coffee beans are the fruit of a plant called the coffee cherry, a type of stone fruit. The fruit is either dried or pulped to release the beans inside the fruit. These are prepared and then roasted.

According to the National Coffee Association, two-thirds of Americans drink coffee daily, making it one of the most popular beverages in the United States. With so many people drinking coffee daily, it's good to know that the DGAs affirm that coffee can be part of a healthy diet. The DGAs support moderate coffee consumption, defined as providing up to 400 mg per day of caffeine. This is the amount in about three to five 8-oz cups.

Many studies have investigated the health benefits of coffee. An article in the March 2018 issue of *Today's Dietitian* Magazine highlights some of these potential health benefits. These include:

- bioactive compounds that have beneficial antioxidant properties
- lower risk of developing type 2 diabetes

- lower incidence of certain types of cancer
- lower risk of developing liver disease
- lower risk of developing or dying from cardiovascular disease

There are some cautions with coffee. Some people may be adversely affected by caffeine and need to limit intake. This includes people with anxiety, high blood pressure, sleep issues, GERD (gastroesophageal reflux disease), and pregnant women.

According to the DGAs, if you are not a coffee drinker, you don't have to begin drinking coffee. Beneficial antioxidants are found in many other plant foods.

Alcohol

Alcohol provides calories, but unlike the other calorie contributing macronutrients—carbohydrates, proteins, and fat—alcohol is not an essential nutrient. Carbohydrates and protein provide 4 calories per gram, fat provides 9 calories per gram, and alcohol provides 7 calories per gram.

While much research has been done regarding the health benefits of alcohol, particularly wine, the DGAs don't recommend that you begin to drink alcohol if you are not currently a drinker.

In fact, the DGAs spell out those who should not drink at all. These include:

- pregnant women
- those under the legal age for drinking
- those taking medications that interact with alcohol
- those who are recovering from alcohol use disorder, or if they are unable to control the amount they drink

Always check with your physician or pharmacist about medications and alcohol interactions. According to the DGAs, if adults ages 21 years and older choose to drink alcohol, there are guidelines. Adults of legal drinking age are recommended to only drink in moderation.

Moderation is defined as:

- 2 drinks or less per day for men
- 1 drink or less per day for women

The following count as one alcoholic drink equivalent:

- 12 fluid ounces of regular beer (5% alcohol)
- 5 fluid ounces of wine (12% alcohol)
- 1.5 fluid ounces of 80 proof distilled spirits (40% alcohol)

This is strictly how much is considered healthy in a day. It is not intended as an average over several days, but rather the amount consumed on any single day. Many people ask if this amount can be saved up and consumed on a weekend or special occasion. No, unfortunately not. Binge drinking is dangerous and should be avoided. Binge drinking is defined as 5 or more drinks for the typical adult male or 4 or more drinks for the typical adult female in about 2 hours.

There is emerging evidence that suggests that even drinking within the recommended limits may increase the overall risk of death from various causes, such as from several types of cancer and some forms of cardiovascular disease. For some types of cancer, the risk increases even at low levels of alcohol consumption (less than 1 drink in a day). Therefore, caution is recommended.

What you choose to drink can make a significant difference, calorie-wise. Here is the calorie content of some common drinks:

- Regular beer (12 oz.) – 150-200
- Light beer (12 oz.) – 95-125
- Wine (5 oz.) – 90-120
- Margarita (8 oz) – 280
- Pina Colada (6 oz) – 378

Dig Deeper

Reflection and action:
1. Examine your tea, coffee, and alcohol habits. Is your consumption within the recommended guidelines?

2. If you are overconsuming, set SMARTER goals to stay within the guidelines, especially for caffeine and alcohol.

Resources and reading:
1. Thalheimer, J.C. (2018). The power of coffee. *Today's Dietitian*, 20(3) 20. https://www.todaysdietitian.com/newarchives/0318p20.shtml

TIP 35 - FIBER FOR FULLNESS AND SO MUCH MORE

"Beans, beans, the musical fruit
The more you eat, the more you toot,
The more you toot, the better you feel.
So, let's have beans for every meal."

Author Unknown

F iber is the structural part of plants and is found in vegetables, fruits, whole grains, legumes, and nuts. It is only found in plant foods. Dietary fibers are similar to starches, but we don't have enzymes to digest them and use them as calories like we do for starches. Some fibers are fermented by intestinal bacteria to produce beneficial probiotics.

Although there is no formal Recommended Dietary Allowance (RDA) for fiber, the Institute for Medicine recommendations for adults include:

- 38 grams per day for men ages 50 years or younger
- 25 grams per day for women ages 50 years or younger
- 30 grams per day for men over 50 years
- 21 grams per day for women over 50 years

Unfortunately, most Americans only get about half of the recommended intake. Some of the benefits of fiber include:

- feeling of fullness and addition of bulk in the diet; this assists with digestion and elimination
- better weight control because you feel full sooner
- prevention of constipation and improved regularity
- prevention or treatment of diverticulosis, diabetes, heart disease, and colon cancer

It's important to increase fiber gradually to help your digestive system adjust. A gradual increase will help decrease gas and diarrhea. Since some fibers absorb water, it's important to increase water intake while increasing fiber. If you continue to have trouble digesting fiber, consider trying an over-the-counter digestive aid, after talking with your healthcare provider.

Remember, all plant foods have some fiber. Whole grains, fruit, vegetables, beans and lentils, and nuts all provide fiber. The DGAs recommend that half of our grains be whole grains. Whole grains contain the full grain that refined grains do not. Refined grains, such as white flour, are enriched with vitamins and minerals to contain similar amounts of vitamins and minerals, but the fiber that is taken out is not added back. Surprisingly, 98% of adults in the U.S. fall below this whole grain recommendation.

Fiber amounts are required by the Food and Drug Administration (FDA) to be included on food labels. This makes it easy to compare fiber content among various brands of breads, crackers, cereals, etc.

In general, individual foods within a food group provide a similar range of fiber, even though the exact amount varies from food to food. Some average ranges are listed below. For a more complete list of the amount of fiber in common foods, see the link in the Dig Deeper section.

- fruits: 2-4 grams per serving (1 medium piece or ½-1 cup)
- vegetables: 2 grams per serving (½ cup cooked or 1 cup raw)
- beans: 7 grams per ½ cup serving cooked
- whole grains, such as pasta, breads, or cereals: 3-10 grams per serving
- nuts: 3 grams per ounce

Dig Deeper

Reflection and action:

1. How much fiber are you getting in a day? Write down everything you eat in a day or two, and then calculate the fiber intake. You can enter it into an app like MyFitnessPal, use the estimates above, or look up the fiber in your food using the Food Sources of Dietary Fiber in the DGAs below.

Resources and reading:

1. Seale, S.A., Sherard, T., & Fleming, D. (2010). *The full plate diet.* Bard Press.

2. Rolls, B. & Hermann, M. (2012). *The ultimate volumetrics diet: Smart, simple, science-based strategies for losing weight and keeping it off.* William Morrows Cookbooks.

3. Dietary fiber in common foods - https://www.dietaryguidelines.gov/resources/2020-2025-dietary-guidelines-online-materials/food-sources-select-nutrients/food-0

TIP 36 - HOW TO BE SLIM BY DESIGN

"The best diet is the one you don't know you're on."

Brian Wansink, author and founder, Family Meal Foundation

Did you know it's important where you keep food in your kitchen? Do you have food on the counter in plain view? On my counter, I used to keep clear glass jars filled with snack foods, such as crackers, nuts, or pretzels. That changed after I read the book *Slim by Design* by Brian Wansink. This interesting book reports on innovative research from the Cornell Food and Brand Lab. For example, their research showed that people eat about 25% less total calories per day if they removed all the visible food in the kitchen, except for a fruit bowl, filled with 1 or 2 types of fruit. Fruit consumption increased with this change. Since most Americans don't eat enough fruit, this is a win-win. In other words, keep fresh fruit in sight and store other foods out of sight. Food in sight, is on your mind. Food out of sight, is out of your mind.

Brian Wansink and team researched how inexpensive design changes, from home kitchens and restaurants to grocery stores and schools or workplaces, can make it mindlessly easy for people to eat healthier. He promotes working WITH human nature instead of AGAINST it.

Some of my favorite tips from his research include:

1. Clear your kitchen counter, except for a full fruit bowl with two or more types of fruit.

2. Drink from taller, thinner glass to help you drink less, including thinner wine glasses.

3. Eat from smaller plates to help you eat less. In fact, Dr. Wansink's research is responsible for the recommendation to eat from a smaller 9-10" plate.

4. You will be satisfied with smaller portions of chocolate, apple pie, or chips than you think. Researchers gave one group of study participants standard servings of the above foods, and another group received a couple of bites of these snack foods. Fifteen minutes later both groups were equally satisfied and happy. The key here is to allow that time to pass after eating.

5. Keep the TV off during meals.

6. Keep pre-cut fruits and vegetables on the center shelf in your refrigerator.

7. Use clear containers to store cut fruit and vegetables.

8. Cereal bowls are best when smaller than 16 ounces.

9. Water glasses are best when 16 ounces or larger.

10. Juice glasses should be 8 ounces or smaller.

11. Eat dinner in the kitchen or at a dining room table.

12. Always keep a glass of water with you.

13. Eat snacks out of small bowls and not out of bags or original containers.

14. Play soft music and dim the lights during dinner to help you eat less.

15. When snacking, keep wrappers of eaten food in sight. This is called the pistachio effect: when you can see the pistachio shells or snack wrappers, it helps you to eat less.

Incorporate these tips and you will improve your eating habits with skill power, and you won't need as much willpower. These tips help to make the healthy choice the easy choice.

Dig Deeper

Reflection and action:

1. Review the layout of your kitchen. Are there things you can change to help you make the healthy choice also the easy choice?

2. Plan to incorporate at least one of the skills listed above over the next week.

Resources and reading:

1. Wansink, B. (2014). *Slim by design: Mindless eating solutions for everyday life.* William Morrow.

TIP 37 - LEARN KITCHEN SAFETY
AND COOK CONFIDENTLY

"When in doubt, throw it out."

Author Unknown

The Centers for Disease Control and Safety estimate there are about 48 million cases of food borne illness every year. According to the Food and Drug Administration (FDA), a foodborne illness is a costly, sometimes life threatening, yet largely preventable, public health problem. Symptoms range from mild to life threatening.

Many outbreaks and individual cases of foodborne illness result from consuming the two most common types of foodborne pathogens. The first is bacteria like salmonella, listeria, or E coli (Escherichia coli). The second is viruses, such as norovirus or hepatitis.

A critical part of healthy eating is keeping food safe. But how? The Partnership for Food Safety Education develops and promotes effective education programs to reduce foodborne illness risk for consumers. Four basic food safety principles work together to reduce the risk of foodborne illness: clean, separate, cook, and chill. These four principles are the cornerstones of their public health campaign Fight BAC!® The following information is taken from Fight BAC!®. Their website is included in the Dig Deeper section.

CLEAN

1. **Wash hands with soap and water**
   Wet hands with clean running water and apply soap. Use warm water if it is available. Rub hands together

to make a lather and scrub all parts of the hand for 20 seconds. (Hum the Happy Birthday song twice). Rinse hands thoroughly and dry using a clean paper towel. If possible, use a clean paper towel to turn off the faucet.

2. **Sanitize surfaces**
   Wash surfaces with hot, soapy water. A solution of 1 tablespoon of unscented, liquid chlorine bleach per gallon of water can be used to sanitize surfaces.

3. **Clean sweep refrigerated foods once a week**
   At least once a week, throw out refrigerated foods that should no longer be eaten. Cooked leftovers should be discarded after four days.

4. **Keep appliances clean**
   Clean the inside and outside of appliances. Pay particular attention to buttons and handles where cross-contamination to hands can occur.

5. **Rinse produce**
   Rinse fresh vegetables and fruits under running water just before eating, cutting, or cooking. Even if you plan to peel or cut the produce before eating, it is important to thoroughly rinse it first to prevent microbes from transferring from the outside to the inside of the produce.

SEPARATE

1. **Separate foods when shopping**
   Place raw seafood, meat, and poultry in plastic bags. Store them below ready-to-eat foods in your refrigerator.

2. **Separate foods when preparing and serving**
   Always use a clean cutting board for fresh produce and a separate one for raw seafood, meat, and poultry.

Never place cooked food back on the same plate or cutting board that previously held raw food.

COOK AND CHILL

1. **Use a food thermometer when cooking**
   A food thermometer should be used to ensure that food is safely cooked and that cooked food is held at safe temperatures until eaten.

2. **Cook food to safe internal temperatures**
   When cooking, check the internal temperature of seafood, meat, poultry, and egg dishes. Cook all raw beef, pork, lamb, and veal steaks, chops, and roasts to a safe minimum internal temperature of 145° F. For safety and quality, allow meat to rest for at least 3 minutes before carving or eating. If the meat is ground, cook all raw ground beef, pork, lamb, and veal to an internal temperature of 160° F. Cook all poultry, including ground turkey and chicken, to an internal temperature of 165° F.

3. **Keep foods at safe temperatures**
   Hold cold foods at 40° F or below. Keep hot foods at 140° F or above. Foods are no longer safe to eat when they have been in the danger zone between 40-140° F for more than 2 hours (1 hour if the temperature was above 90° F).

How Long to Keep Food

I highly recommend the USDA FoodKeeper app for the most complete list of safe storage times. It provides guidance on the safe handling, preparation, and storage of food. The app offers specific storage timelines for the refrigerator, freezer, and pantry for most food items. It offers cooking tips and methods for meat, poultry, and seafood. Products can be added to a calendar for you to receive notifications when they are nearing the end of their recommended storage date. You will receive information on food safety recalls. You can search for foods in English, Spanish, and Portuguese. The app is available for Android and Apple. You can also access it online.

Dig Deeper

Reflection and action:

1. Reviewing the habits above, what areas need improvement in your life for better food safety?

2. Keep a thermometer in your refrigerator and freezer to remove any guesswork about the temperatures inside.

3. Use a thermometer when cooking meat, poultry, and fish to ensure safe cooking temperatures are reached.

4. Remember to keep foods in safe temperature ranges when on a picnic or cookout. Serving dishes with ice are great for serving foods. Coolers with ice are great to store foods before and after eating.

Resources and reading:

1. The Partnership for Food Safety Education - https://www.fightbac.org/

2. The FoodKeeper App and Website - https://www.foodsafety.gov/keep-food-safe/foodkeeper-app

POEM - THE DIET RIOT

I wrote this poem in the wee hours of the morning after watching a panel of physicians testifying before Congress about the upcoming Dietary Guidelines for Americans. They all had different beliefs about what constitutes a healthy diet. I was awake watching until about 2 a.m., glued to the arguments each distinguished physician passionately believed and promoted.

❋ ❋ ❋

The Diet Riot
By Theresa Yosuico Stahl

I eagerly searched for the perfect diet,
but what I found was a diet riot.
High-protein, high-carb: the diet gurus
dish out diet advice telling me what to do.
And they all disagree, and they love to debate.
And while they discuss, I'm gaining more weight.
So please diet gurus, get your information straight
because I need a diet, and this just can't wait.

Well, maybe…
If I'd eat healthy food from sunrise to bed
and not overstuff till I feel like I'm dead.
And have my diet analyzed by a registered dietitian
and take that advice as my eating prescription
and drink plenty of water and get enough rest
and exercise daily - I'd feel at my best.
Maybe then I'd be done with those diets for life
and the diet riot wouldn't cause me such strife.
I'd be healthy as can be from my head to my toes
And be done, once and for all, with my dieting woes.

PART THREE- TIPS TO MANAGE STRESS AND IMPROVE MOOD

* * *

TIP 38 - HARNESS THE POWER OF YOUR THOUGHTS AND WORDS

"All things be ready if our minds be so."

William Shakespeare

The words we speak have power. Have you ever heard the toothpaste analogy about words? It goes something like this: The teacher asked a child to squeeze out some toothpaste. Next, they were asked to put it back. The lesson: Our words are like toothpaste. Once you say them, you cannot take them back. Please be careful with what you say and choose your words wisely. Words begin with thoughts. If we can control our thoughts, we can better control our words and actions.

Often, we are our own worst critics. Especially when it comes to eating habits. Have you ever been your own worst critic? Unfortunately, many of our thoughts are thought distortions or distorted thoughts. This means they are not true, but we tell them to ourselves or hear them in our head and choose to believe them.

Here are some examples of thought distortions:

- "Oh, go ahead and eat more cake, you already blew your diet anyway and you know it tastes so good and you want it."
- "Tomorrow I start my diet, so tonight I am going to eat all of my favorites for the last time."
- "I can't do this. I have tried to eat healthy before, but I never stick with it. I have no willpower."
- "I look awful...I'm too fat."

Have you ever said any of these to yourself or heard these messages in your mind? These are destructive thoughts. This distorted thinking interferes with your best efforts to achieve your goals. Remember, if you would not talk to your friend or your family this way, then why talk to yourself this way? The Golden Rule—Do unto others as you would have them do unto you—applies here as well. We need to treat ourselves with the same kindness and respect that we give to others.

Kindness Matters

The kindness we show to others, and the kindness we show to ourselves matters. Instead of being your own worst enemy, why not be your own best friend? It is not easy to make these kinds of changes in your thought life. Imagine a STOP sign as a mental symbol and use this visual as soon as negative, critical thoughts begin. STOP the negative self-talk. The sooner you put a stop to these negative thoughts, the sooner you can move forward in your quest to be healthy and achieve your goals. Encourage your-self as you would your best friend or your child. You are worth it.

Here are some ways to reframe thought distortions:

- "If I overate and now feel stuffed, I will be more mindful and pay more attention next time. I will eat more slowly and savor each bite to prevent this from happening again."
- "I am making healthy choices most of the time. It is all right to enjoy my favorite treats once in a while, too"
- "I can do this."
- "I can enjoy chocolate in moderation."

Try to think happy thoughts. A wooden sign with these words hangs in my office. It reminds me of the importance of my thoughts and reminds me that what I think about becomes a conscious decision. As Walt Disney said, "Whether you say you can't or you can, you're right." Our thoughts are powerful. Our words are powerful.

<u>Dig Deeper</u>

Reflection and action:

1. What thought distortions do you tell yourself? Write them down and reframe them into healthy thoughts. Use the examples above, if desired.

Resources and reading:

1. Karen Salmansohn's website and books -
www.notsalmon.com

2. Newberry, T. (2007). *The 4:8 Principle: The Secret to a Joy-Filled Life.* Tyndale.

TIP 39 - BE BALANCED AND MODERATE

"We should have open minds, but not so
open that our brains fall out."

Attributed to many different authors

B alance is defined as a happy medium, moderation, and a state of stability resulting from the cancellation of all forces by equal opposing forces. Balanced is defined as sane, clear headed, and undisturbed.

According to a 2019 report, "The U.S. Weight Loss and Diet Control Market," it is estimated that Americans spend over $72 billion per year in the weight loss market. Yet, rates of obesity continue to rise in the United States. According to a report in *The New England Journal of Medicine*, the current generation may have a shorter life expectancy than their parents.

Too often, moderation in food intake is being replaced with extreme and misguided thinking about nutrition. For example, while some people require a gluten-free diet due to celiac disease or non-celiac gluten sensitivity, many are deleting the wheat to lose weight or simply because they heard gluten was bad.

People go to extremes to lose weight. One future bride went as far as to go on a tube feeding to control her calorie intake and lose weight for her wedding. Why are people so extreme about eating habits?

Could it be nutrition information overload? Have you ever felt that you do not know what to believe? Have you ever felt anxious about eating? It is normal to want to keep up with the latest nutrition research, but it's best to seek nutrition advice from a qualified nutrition professional. Some people become so anxious about eating that they develop a condition called orthorexia. Symptoms include an obsession with eating only foods that one considers to be healthy, while avoiding foods perceived to be unhealthy. In severe cases, this can lead to death.

Balance Is Lost

Why is balance lost? If you have had to deal with a lack of food at some point in your life, you may subconsciously fear that each meal may be your last. This often occurs in people who have lived through the Great Depression or poverty or even a history of dieting.

Some people are so sick of dieting and restricting foods, that their pendulum swings the other way. They know that the dieting industry has had it wrong. But instead of achieving healthy eating habits and balance, they give up caring about what they eat and often their health suffers.

Regaining Balance

Through my client work, I know many people gravitate toward extreme diets. Yet, for some, even just the word diet evokes feelings of deprivation. If you feel deprived every day, this may lead to more unhealthy habits. Healthy eating is not about deprivation. It's about healthy habits.

Be Moderate

How can you balance the scales with your own eating habits? How can you stick with a healthy diet without having to say "no" to your favorite treats and without feeling deprived? You don't have to give up your favorite treats. It's all about how much and how frequently.

- Eat healthy, nutrient-rich foods most of the time. You do not have to be on a diet to eat healthy. Just say "I am choosing to eat healthy." This will eliminate the whole "diet" and "deprivation" mentality that can lead to binge eating.

- Enjoy less healthy favorites less frequently and in

small amounts. Learn to eat mindfully by focusing on enjoying each bite and you'll be satisfied with less. Remember, research shows the greatest satisfaction comes from the first few bites.

- If you feel stumped about how to do this, meet with a registered dietitian nutritionist who can give you specific pointers on how to fit in your favorite splurge foods.

The Power of Permission

The more you deprive yourself of your favorite foods, the more you desire them. Deprivation leads to bingeing, sneaking food, guilt, and shame. There's no reason for this. It's a vicious cycle. There's something in human nature, for some more than others, that tends toward "all or nothing" or "black and white" thinking. You are either on a diet or off a diet. You are either being "good" or being "bad." These people tend to love the "eat this not that" form of eating. "Just tell me what to eat," they say. "Eat real food, mostly plants, and not too much." This famous advice from Michael Pollan's book, *Food Rules*, sums up basic, scientifically-sound eating advice.

"Balance, variety, and moderation," has been the mantra of the Academy of Nutrition and Dietetics since I began studying nutrition in the late 1970s. Balance your plate with foods from each food group. Eat a variety of foods within each food group. And eat in moderation (not too much). Following mindful eating principles help you eat as much as you need, and not too much. This advice seems to elude some people because of "all or nothing" thinking. This is a form of distorted thinking that some people call "stinking thinking."

How can you give yourself permission to enjoy your favorite foods, even if they are high calorie and low nutritional value? The secret is twofold: how frequently you eat them and how much of them you eat are the keys!

As I've said before, I love ice cream. But how frequently I eat it and how much I eat when I do are the keys to helping me enjoy it in moderation and maintain a healthy weight and balance in my eating habits. I also love fried food, but it doesn't love me back, so how frequently I eat it and how much I eat is key to feeling my best. I love chocolate, but how frequently I eat it and how much I eat is key to helping me maintain my weight.

This helps in the most practical ways. For example, I discovered an ice cream treat that I really liked. I began eating it but soon I was eating it every night and began looking forward to it every day. Sure enough, the scale began creeping up. I like to maintain my weight within a certain range, rather than trying to stay at a certain number on the scale. This is more practical, as weights go up and down and being too strict can become obsessive. So, when I see my weight creeping up to the top of my desired weight range, I "tighten up" on my eating habits. I realized that adding that ice cream treat every night did not work. I decided to eliminate it, but I could have just as easily decided to eat it only once or twice a week and then reexamine how it was impacting me. I think I ate enough of it to satisfy me for a while and I didn't like the "addictive" nature of it, so I just let it go. In doing that, I lost my desire for it.

Dark chocolate, on the other hand, is not something I want to give up entirely. It has many health benefits, so I include a small piece or two about 3-5 days per week. This doesn't interfere with maintaining my healthy weight range. But if I begin to eat several pieces every day, then my weight would creep up. Some of my clients don't like to keep chocolate in the house, saying it will call their name until the bag is gone. We are all individuals and each of us must decide how much and how frequently works for us.

As I mentioned before, an order of onion rings may provide about 400 calories but shared between four people, only 100 calories each. I can satisfy my desire for fried foods in a reasonable way. I don't feel I'm depriving myself of my fried food favorites. As an alternative, many people are enjoying the air fryer as a healthier alternative to deep frying, with the same crunchy satisfaction.

These are a few examples from my own firsthand experiences. How you stay balanced and moderate will be unique to you since we're all different. This tip creates a win-win situation. You and I enjoy our favorite treats without blowing our health goals. The power of permission destroys feelings of deprivation and enhances enjoyment of some favorite foods.

Dig Deeper

Reflection and action:

1. Do you deprive yourself of some of your favorite foods? Could you plan to include them? How often or how much?

Resources and reading:

1. The Moderation Movement - www.moderationmovement.com.au

2. The U.S. Weight Loss and Diet Control Market at the Research and Markets online store - https:// www.researchandmarkets.com/research/qm2gts/ the_72_billion?w=4

3. Olshansky, S. Passaro, D., Hershow, R., Layden, J., Carnes, B., Brody, J., Hayflick, L., Butler, R., Allison, D., & Ludwig, D. (2005). A potential decline in life expectancy in the United States in the 21st century. *The New England Journal of Medicine*. Massachusetts Medical Society. https://doi.org/10.1056/NEJMsr043743

TIP 40 - STRESS LESS

"Desserts is stressed spelled backwards."

Author Unknown

Accoording to an article in the *Journal of the American Medical Association*, 60-80% of visits to primary care provider offices are related to stress. Yet only 3% receive any counseling about stress management, including referrals for help with their stress.

As a registered dietitian nutritionist (RDN), I help people improve their eating habits to feel their best and manage or prevent chronic diseases such as hypertension, hyperlipidemia, heart disease, and type 2 diabetes. Stress is a significant factor in health and affects chronic diseases. In fact, stress can be a factor in every area of health—physical, mental, emotional, spiritual, and behavioral.

Some stress is positive, and some is negative. The positive stress, called eustress, propels us forward. We feel we can handle this type of stress, and we rise to the occasion to conquer daily obstacles. It feels manageable.

Negative stress, or distress, feels overwhelming and too much to handle. This stress, via the sympathetic nervous system, triggers a cascade of physical changes in our body known as fight or flight. Can you relate? For example, your child (or friend) is about to run into the street in front of a car and you rush as fast as you can to save him. Your adrenaline kicks in. Your blood pressure and blood sugar rise. Cortisol is released to kick start you into action. Your digestion is halted to allow all your energy to empower your muscles to reach your child (or friend) before any harm befalls her. Afterward, your body returns to normal. Homeostasis or balance returns. But sometimes, after multiple or prolonged stresses, your body can become stuck or freezes. This is where health problems may occur.

Our autonomic nervous system plays a key role in our stress response. People once believed the autonomic nervous system was automatic. For example, you don't need to consciously make your heartbeat or digest your food. These are automatic. But much research has demonstrated that we have more control over our body's responses than originally believed. Parts of our autonomic nervous system include the sympathetic and para-sympathetic nervous systems

The antidote to the "fight or flight" response is the activation of our parasympathetic nervous system, our "rest and digest" system. By deep breathing and other mindful practices, we acti-vate our vagus nerve that releases the hormones serotonin and oxytocin. These hormones help bring us back into balance and connect with others better. Our blood pressure and heart rates improve.

As I write this, we are in the midst of the global COVID-19 pandemic. Civil unrest, political discord, and natural disasters abound. Increased stress is having an effect on all of us. How we respond influences our health.

If your eating habits tend to get out of balance when you're stressed, then you're not alone. Unfortunately, many people reach for high-calorie, high-fat, high-sodium, and high-sugar foods when they're stressed. Many of these are ultra-processed foods that have been associated with weight gain and poor health. This may have begun at an early age when a caring par-ent or grandparent gave a cookie for a skinned knee. Or an ice cream cone after a rough day. Turning to food for comfort is a behavior passed down by the most well-intentioned people. But, turning to food or drink for comfort or to manage stress isn't the best way to deal with stress and can create other health issues. For example, if you turn to eating for stress management, the result may be weight gain or elevated blood sugar or blood pressure, and the addition of yet another new stress. Turning to alcohol or sugar-sweetened beverages is not a healthy solution either.

Instead, choose healthy alternatives to manage stress:

1. Exercise helps to increase "feel good" brain chemicals such as serotonin and is one of the best ways to manage daily stress.

2. Regular meals and healthy snacks help to control blood sugar levels, which help promote stable moods instead of the mood swings associated with erratic blood sugar levels.

3. Stay hydrated. Often you may think you're hungry when you're thirsty. Drink water most of the time. Try a slice of fresh fruit in sparkling water for a festive and refreshing drink. Infuse water with herbs, such as mint, and fruits or vegetables, such as cucumbers. More ideas in Tip 33: Rethink Your Drink.

4. Practice mindfulness and meditation. There will be more tips to come related to this topic.

5. Get outside. Being in nature increases our serotonin and improves our health.

After completing the Professional Training in Mind-Body Medicine, I experienced a major shift in thinking about doing the things that make me feel better, such as getting out in nature, deep breathing, meditation, and prayer. The evidence-based research convinced me that there are scientific reasons why I love these things and why I feel so great during and after them. I shifted from doing these things WHEN I had time, to MAKING TIME to do them for better health.

Know When to Say No

In this book, we have talked about a full plate in terms of the food we put on our plate, but there's another interpretation as well. The expression, "My plate is full," also has significance in living a full life. We usually say "my plate is full" when we are too busy to take on another responsibility. For many of us, "our plates are overfull." Just as with our plates of food and our stomachs, overfull is not desirable. Knowing when your plate is full takes skill, mindfulness, and knowing yourself very well. Learning to say no is empowering.

I learned this the hard way. When I was in my early 30s, I became noticeably short of breath one day, so short of breath that I couldn't even stand to fold my laundry. This was unexpected and unheard of for me. Since it was a Friday, I decided to see my doctor and get checked out before the weekend. This was in the days before urgent care clinics. My doctor listened to my chest and immediately ordered a chest x-ray. The news wasn't good. He called that evening, "I need to admit you to the hospital immediately. You either have cancer or sarcoidosis."

"What?"

This news hit like a ton of bricks. My heart sank. Cancer? Sarcoidosis? I had never even heard of sarcoidosis, but it didn't sound like anything I wanted. Yet, it sounded better than cancer, I thought. After a week of daily testing, I got my diagnosis. I had sarcoidosis!

This diagnosis began a new journey for me. In my early 30s with a 4-year-old daughter, an 18-month-old son, and a busy executive husband, I needed to enlist help around my house. I cut back on my part-time work as an RDN in a busy pediatric practice, limited volunteer work, and slowed down.

For me, that was a big challenge and throughout the many years since, life has been a balancing act. If I do too much, I get sick. And then I will be completely down and out for the count.

It was during those early years, when I was the sickest, that I learned the invaluable lesson of saying no. I learned there are many good things to do, but they may not be the best things for me. I had to learn to select what I wanted to do. I had to be flexible with my schedule because sometimes I would have to cancel plans due to my poor health. Life's challenging times teach us many lessons, and this is the lesson I learned during my sickest years. I have carried it with me ever since.

Learning to say no when your plate is full is a beneficial skill for everyone. Sick or not, we risk running ourselves down, weakening our immune systems, increasing our stress, and increasing the likelihood of getting sick. Maintaining a healthy balance in our lives matters for better health.

Dig Deeper

Reflection and action:

1. Were you raised using food as comfort or stress management?

2. What are your current ways of dealing with stress, both healthy and unhealthy?

3. Set SMARTER goals for increasing healthy ways to deal with stress in your life. For example, I will take a relaxing bath in the evening three times a week. Or, I will not agree to a new commitment when asked, instead I will say, "I will think about it and get back to you this week."

Resources and reading:

1. Nerurkar, A., Bitton, A., Davis, R. B., Phillips, R. S., & Yeh, G. (2013). When physicians counsel about stress: results of a national study. *JAMA Internal Medicine, 173*(1), 76–77. https://doi.org/10.1001/2013.jamainternmed.480

2. Fogt, E., & Shah, N. (2014). *Having your all: How self-care leads to an energized, empowered and effective life.* Women Wellness.

TIP 41 - BE MINDFUL

"The best way to capture moments is to pay attention.
This is how we cultivate mindfulness."

Jon Kabat-Zinn, professor, writer, and mindfulness expert

According to the Oxford Dictionary, mindfulness means the quality or state of being conscious or aware of something, and the mental state achieved by focusing one's awareness on the present moment, while calmly acknowledging and accepting one's feelings, thoughts, and bodily sensations. This is used as a therapeutic technique. In short, mindfulness is paying attention to the present.

We can apply mindfulness to many of our daily activities. When used with eating or walking or meditation, it simply means paying attention while doing the activity. In this fast-paced, digital world, we have more distractions than ever. Paying attention seems more difficult. But this is precisely the reason we need to be mindful. As author Anne Lamott writes, "Almost everything will work again if you unplug it for a few minutes, including you." Unfortunately, our culture seems to prize multi-tasking to get as much done in as little time as possible. But this has taken a toll on health. A search on PubMed.gov, the database of the National Institutes of Health's Library of Medicine, reveals over 20,000 citations for journal articles on mindfulness.

Some benefits of mindfulness include:

- improving the quality of life and decreasing mental health symptoms for people with chronic illnesses, such as depression, high blood pressure, diabetes, and heart disease

- supporting healthy immune system function

- helping people manage stress

- improving concentration

- lengthening lives by reducing cell damage

- improving healthy eating habits

Remember, mindful eating includes choosing foods with intention, while also paying attention while eating.

A great visual I have used in many presentations includes a person looking out over a beautiful view with their dog by their side. The person has a thought bubble over their head filled with all the worries of their past, present, and future. The caption for this image is "Mind Full." Beside that image is the same person with a thought bubble overhead with just him and the dog and the view. And the caption for this image is "Mindful."

We truly can be physically present, but mentally all over the place and not really paying attention to the present moment. In order to slow down and appreciate life, one must first notice the roses along the way. Too many times, our minds are wandering and oblivious to the beauty that surrounds us. Mindfulness helps change that by bringing us into the present moment.

I have heard it said that yesterday is history, tomorrow is a mystery, and today is a gift of God, which is why we call it the present. Attributed to Bill Keane, the cartoonist of Family Circus fame, it reminds us to be mindful.

In the upcoming tips, I will review various skills to help you improve your mindfulness. These skills will help you better manage stress and lead to improved health.

<u>Dig Deeper</u>

Reflection and action:

1. Do you live in the present moment or are you often focusing on the past or the future?

2. What could you do to help yourself live in the present moment more frequently?

Resources and reading:

1. Gordon, J.S. (2019). *The Transformation.* Harper One.

TIP 42 - BREATHE DEEPLY

"Change your breathing, change your life."

Author Unknown

From our first cry when we leave our mother's womb and arrive in this world, to our dying breath, breathing is required for life. Breathing is a subconscious act our body performs about 25,000 times a day. I facilitate 8-week, mind-body skills groups to help others learn practical stress management techniques. During one group where we were reviewing deep breathing for stress management, one of my group participants remarked, "I have been breathing my whole life. This is not anything new."

Why make such a fuss about breathing? In medical terminology, the act of taking a breath is called inspiration. In many languages, including Hebrew, Arabic, Greek, Latin, and Sanskrit, the word for breath is synonymous with the word for spirit or life. In the words of the Bible, "Then the Lord God formed a man from the dust of the ground and breathed into his nostrils the breath of life, and the man became a living being." (Genesis)

Breathing, part of the respiratory system, is both involuntary and voluntary. The involuntary part keeps us alive. Most breaths are shallow and short. Voluntarily breathing more slowly and deeply than usual aides in relaxation and stress management which add quality to our lives.

Singers learn deep breathing to sing better. I did not learn deep breathing by singing in a choir; my first experience with deep breathing came during my childbirth classes. Deep breathing is taught to help manage pain during labor and childbirth. My first regular practice of deep breathing came while teaching PraiseMoves, a Christian alternative to yoga, consisting of deep breathing and stretching to scriptures. Deep diaphragmatic breathing was a part of every class, and aides in movement and relaxation.

In our daily lives, most of us are not routinely breathing deeply. According to a 2017 article in the journal *Breathe*, the typical respiratory rate in humans is within the range of 10-20 breaths per minute. Slow breathing (soft belly breathing or deep diaphragmatic breathing) is any rate from 4-10 breaths per minute.

In times of stress, breathing becomes shallower. Ordinarily, your chest rises and falls when you take a breath. But if you take a deeper inspiration, your abdomen rises and falls with more definition. When you breathe deeply into your diaphragm, your abdomen rises first on the in-breath and then your chest rises. They both soften on the out-breath.

Dr. James Gordon, founder and director of the Center for Mind-Body Medicine, calls this "soft-belly breathing." I like that because it is figurative and expresses what happens in the deep breath. It reminds me to soften and focus on my belly, or abdomen, when I breathe. It is only possible when taking your breath deep into your abdomen. This deep breathing helps you relax, lowers your blood pressure, and lowers your heart rate.

Never underestimate the power of the simplest of stress management techniques. One participant in my 12-week nutrition program shared that during his Master of Business Administration studies, one insightful professor taught the class the importance of deep breathing which they practiced during class. He said this deep breathing exercise stuck with him ever since. He said it was one of the most important tools he learned.

Dig Deeper

Reflection and action:

1. Examine your breathing and practice deep breathing throughout the day. Notice the difference in how you feel when you take

time to breathe in slowly and deeply.

2. Practice breathing slowly and deeply in through your nose and out through your mouth for 5 minutes every morning and evening; do it throughout the day when you feel anxious, nervous, or stressed.

Resources and reading:

1. Russo, M. A., Santarelli, D. M., & O'Rourke, D. (2017). The physiological effects of slow breathing in the healthy human. *Breathe,* 13(4), 298-309. https://doi.org/10.1183/20734735.009817

2. Gordon, J.S. (2019). *The Transformation.* Harper One.

TIP 43 - MEDITATE

"Half an hour's meditation each day is essential, except when you are busy. Then a full hour is needed."
Saint Francis De Sales, Bishop of Geneva and author

"And now, dear brothers and sisters, one final thing. Fix your thoughts on what is true, and honorable, and right, and pure, and lovely, and admirable. Think about things that are excellent and worthy of praise."
Philippians 4.8 New Living Translation

What do you think of when you hear the word meditation? I used to think of someone sitting on the floor with their legs crossed, quietly thinking about something intently. I remember my first awareness of meditation came from the Beatles in the late 1960s. John, Paul, George, and Ringo went to India to study transcendental meditation. Photos of the Beatles sitting cross-legged followed. Shortly after, one of my cousins, who was a college student, became the first person I personally knew to begin meditating on a regular basis.

Since then, hundreds of studies have been conducted to assess the health benefits of meditation. One research article published in the *Journal of the American Medical Association* in 2013 reviewed well-designed, reliable studies. Some of the health benefits of meditation that they identified at that time included reducing anxiety, depression, and pain.

Interestingly, the words meditate, and medicine come from the same root word that means to "to care for" or "to take measure of." Meditation changes our brains for the better. It has been shown to lower blood pressure, slow aging and help us think more clearly and feel more connected to people.

According to the Mayo Clinic, "Meditation may offer many benefits, such as helping with concentration, relaxation, inner peace, stress reduction and fatigue. When combined with conventional medicine, meditation may improve physical health. Other research suggests meditation can help manage symptoms of conditions such as insomnia, heart disease, pain, cancer, and digestive problems."

The actor Dick Van Dyke said, "When you're a kid, you lay in the grass and watch the clouds going by and you literally don't have a thought in your mind. It's purely meditation, and we lose that." Do you remember laying in the grass and watching the clouds? I do. I spent many hours doing just that. I remember the wonderful feeling of freedom I felt just watching the clouds roll by. Sometimes, my imagination would run wild looking at those clouds while imagining what I was seeing in those flowing shapes. Pretty amazing. To this day, I enjoy seeing peoples' photos of clouds that resemble angels or other captivating shapes.

According to Dr. James Gordon, there are three major types of meditation. The first is concentrative meditation. This involves focused awareness on a particular object, such as the breath, with deep breathing meditation. Some prayer and focusing on sounds or visual images are also examples of concentrative meditation. Much research has been done on concentrative meditation. Deep, "soft-belly" breathing is a concentrative meditation. I love that the word "breathe" has found its way onto many memes and art objects. It's a welcome reminder when we need it.

The second type of meditation is mindfulness or awareness meditation. This involves being relaxed and aware of your thoughts, feelings, and sensations as they arise. Mindfulness helps us to be present in each moment and to become aware of exactly what we feel and see in each moment. Mindful walking helps us to be more observant on our walks. Mindful eating helps us to fully savor the flavor of our food and may help us to become more satisfied eating less food. We are encouraged to use this type of meditation when we are told to "stop and smell the roses" or "slow down and savor the flavor of our food."

The third type of meditation is expressive meditation, such as dancing, shaking, chanting, rapid breathing, and whirling. This helps to break up stuck patterns in our bodies such as negative fixed ideas, and feelings of grief, anger, and despair. It also helps to disperse nervous energy. I wish I had learned about this type of meditation when I was child. My mom would often say to me, "What's the matter with you? Do you have ants in your pants? Can't you sit still?" The truth was, I struggled with sitting still. I had a lot of energy. My mom wisely enrolled me in tap and ballet classes to help expend some of that endless energy. I often wish I had learned about shaking as a child.

Expressive meditation helps bring stillness and awareness after extreme activity. Think about how well you sleep after an exhilarating and active day. When someone encourages you to "shake the jitters or your sillies out," they are encouraging this type of meditation. Along with prayer, this is my "go-to meditation" before I teach a class, webinar, or record a video. It shakes out the nervousness and brings a relaxed calm that helps me focus better.

It's great to have many forms of meditation to meet the different situations in our daily lives. I try to use concentrative, mindfulness, and expressive meditations daily. The more you practice, the quicker they become part of your everyday life.

There are many excellent books on meditation and apps that help with meditation. I will include some below for you to explore. I use them all at various times. Sometimes a guided meditation is just what I need. Besides the apps listed below, there are many free examples of meditation available on YouTube.com.

Take time to make meditation part of your everyday life. You will be better for it.

Dig Deeper

Reflection and action:

1. Do you have a regular meditation practice?

2. If not, write a SMARTER goal to incorporate some form of meditation daily. For example, I will breathe deeply for 5 minutes each day.

Resources and reading:

1. Gordon, J.S. (2019). *The Transformation.* Harper One.

2. The Center for Mind-Body Medicine – www.cmbm.org - free meditations to practice under the heading "education" under the "self-care resources" and free webinars under the "webinars" heading in that same section.

3. Insight Timer App – www.insighttimer.com

4. Calm App – www.calm.com

5. Abide Bible and Meditation App – https://abide.co/

6. Nerurkar, A., Bitton, A., Davis, R. B., Phillips, R. S., & Yeh, G. (2013). When physicians counsel about stress: results of a national study. *JAMA Internal Medicine, 173*(1), 76–77. https://doi.org/10.1001/2013.jamainternmed.480

TIP 44 - LAUGH

"A happy heart is good medicine, and a cheerful mind works healing."

Proverbs 17.22 (Amplified Bible)

"The human race has one really effective weapon and that is laughter."

Mark Twain, American writer

I love to laugh. I've been known to laugh at inappropriate times. At funerals, in class, while on the phone. It's embarrassing, really. I've been doing it for as long as I can remember. Once it starts, it's difficult to stop.

Sometimes my laughing has gotten me in trouble. I remember being in 8th grade in Catholic school, with an extremely strict nun. Something silly struck me as funny and I began laughing. A couple of my friends, sitting around me, joined in. The more we tried to stop, the harder we laughed. The laughter continued until we all got in trouble for our "uncontrolled" behavior, and it was back to reality.

I completed my certification in mind-body medicine through the Center for Mind-Body Medicine in Washington, D.C. While I was taking part in my certification training program, I was in a group with a physician who explained to our group that the best and most complete exhale occurs during a strong belly laugh. Knowing what we know about the health benefits of deep breathing, laughing is a fun way to take some deep breaths.

There are many health benefits of laughter. Here are some:

- stimulates organs by enhancing your intake of oxygen-rich air, laughter stimulates your heart, lungs, and muscles, and increases the endorphins that are released by your brain

- activates and relieves stress response

- may decrease pain and anxiety

- soothes tension by stimulating circulation and aiding in muscle relaxation, both of which can help reduce some of the physical symptoms of stress

- improves the immune system by helping to release neuropeptides that help fight stress

- increases personal satisfaction by helping us better cope with demanding situations and to connect with other people

- improves mood

Even when life is challenging, which often seems like every day, find reasons to laugh. Turn off the news and turn on a comedy. Spend time with people who make you laugh. I'm guilty of taking myself too seriously. Are you? I am working on changing that and am attempting to laugh at myself more often.

Dig Deeper

Reflection and action:

1. When was the last time you had a deep belly laugh?

2. Write a SMARTER goal to help you be intentional about adding more laughter into your life. For example, I will watch a light-hearted comedy skit or show every week.

Resources and reading:

1. *Mayo Clinic.* Stress Relief from Laughter? It's No Joke. https://www.mayoclinic.org/healthy-lifestyle/stress-management/in-depth/stress-relief/art-20044456

TIP 45 - SLEEP

"Sleep is the best meditation."
Dalai Lama

"No day is so bad it can't be fixed with a nap."
Carrie Snow, writer and comedian

Before I learned about the connection between sleep and health, I envied people who didn't seem to need much sleep. Didn't they get more accomplished? But in recent years, research shows the importance of sleep for health and longevity. Now I admire people who make sleep a priority.

Following a 12-month project conducted by a Consensus Panel of 15 of the nation's foremost sleep experts, the American Academy of Sleep Medicine and the Sleep Research Society recommends at least seven hours of sleep as optimum to avoid the health risks of inadequate sleep. Interestingly, they did not put a limit on the upper hours of recommended sleep.

Although you are unconscious during sleep, your brain and your body are still quite active helping you stay healthy and function at your best. Sleeping at least seven hours per night helps support a healthy immune system and decreases risk for heart attack. Not getting enough sleep is linked to increased risk of obesity and diabetes.

According to a study by the Centers for Disease Control and Prevention (CDC), more than 30% of American adults aren't getting enough sleep (less than seven hours per night) to function at their best. Part of my nutrition assessment is asking clients about their sleep habits. Early in my career, I was surprised by how many obese clients had trouble sleeping. But as research has emerged about the connection between sleep and weight, I am no longer surprised.

Overweight and obesity are also linked with the medical diagnosis of sleep apnea. Sleep apnea causes your breathing to stop or get very shallow. Breathing pauses can last from a few seconds to minutes and may occur 30 times or more an hour. The most common type is obstructive sleep apnea. It causes your airway to collapse or become blocked during sleep. Normal breathing starts again with a snort or choking sound. People with sleep apnea often snore loudly. It is important to note that not everyone who snores has sleep apnea. Risk for sleep apnea increases if you are overweight or obese, male, have a family history, or have small airways.

As mentioned, sleep is an important piece in the weight control puzzle. We most often think of calorie intake and exercise as being the main players. Stress management plays an important role as well. I often use the illustration of a pyramid with calorie intake, exercise, and stress management as the three sides of the pyramid. Sleep falls into the stress management side.

Not only do studies reveal that people who get less than seven hours of sleep per night have a higher incidence of obesity, but the rate of obesity also increases as the hours of sleep decrease. One factor has to do with the hormones, leptin and ghrelin. Ghrelin is the hormone associated with hunger and leptin is the hormone associated with fullness. If you don't get enough sleep, your ghrelin levels rise, and your leptin levels decrease. This means you are hungrier, and you don't feel your fullness as well. This may promote overeating. Have you ever noticed when you aren't sleeping well, you crave more food and less healthy food? I have personally noticed this. Making sleep a priority can help you achieve or maintain a healthier weight.

How can you improve your sleep?

- Daily movement during the day can help with sleep. Any movement is better than none, but 30-60 minutes is a good goal. Limit vigorous movement too close to bedtime, though, as it might be stimulating.

- Use your bedroom mainly for sleep and not for watching TV or working.

- Limit caffeine intake, especially later in the day and evening.

- Limit alcohol intake because alcohol-induced sleep isn't restful sleep.

- Limit late night fluid intake to decrease nighttime awakenings due to the need to urinate.

- Don't go to bed too hungry or too full because either extreme can interfere with sleep.

- Enjoy a nightly routine.

- Dim the lights to help prepare your body for sleep.

- Turn off screens or unplug for at least one-half hour before bed.

- If you are not able to sleep for an extended period of time, consider seeing a sleep specialist.

Dig Deeper

Reflection and action:

1. Examine your own sleep habits. Are you getting at least seven hours of sleep consistently?

2. If not, what can you do to improve your sleep habits? Set a SMARTER goal about how you will improve your sleep habits. For example, I will read before bed for one half-hour, instead of watching TV, for 4-5 nights per week.

Resources and reading:

1. American Academy of Sleep Medicine – www.aasm.org

2. Sleep Education – www.sleepeducation.org

TIP 46 - MOVEMENT AND EXERCISE

"Exercise not only changes your body, but it also
changes your attitude and your mood."

Author Unknown

D o you enjoy exercise? Do you think it's fun, or do you view it as punishment for eating too many calories, or as permission to eat extra calories? I've learned that many people think negatively of exercise, often stemming way back to gym classes in school. Instead of thinking of exercise, think of it as movement. I've heard it referred to as joyful movement. I think exercise should be fun and playful.

We are made to move. Research reveals it is harmful to our bodies when we don't. Have you heard it said that "Sitting is the new smoking?" This is because there is cardiovascular damage from too much sitting.

Benefits of Movement and Exercise

1. Improves mood – Exercise increases serotonin, our happy hormone, and decreases cortisol, our stress hormone. And we usually just feel good about ourselves after exercising. We know we've done something good for ourselves which boosts self-esteem.

2. Improves blood pressure – Exercise has been shown to lower blood pressure, thus helping to prevent or manage hypertension.

3. Improves blood sugar – Exercise works like medicine to help our bodies use insulin which helps to regulate blood sugar levels. So, exercise helps to prevent or manage type 2 diabetes. And it helps manage type 1 diabetes.

4. Improves bone health – Weight bearing exercise, including hiking, brisk walking, yoga, tai chi, lifting weights, among others, help to keep bones strong and prevent osteoporosis. Osteoporosis, or thinning bones, makes one more likely to fracture bones. This disease is often associated with women and aging, but men can develop osteoporosis, too.

5. Improves sleep – Research has shown that exercise improves sleep. I must say that I have noticed this benefit in my own life, but I must be careful not to do vigorous exercise too close to bedtime. It may give you more energy (another benefit) and make it harder to fall asleep. Exercise, not too close to bedtime, is one of the best things I can do for a good night's sleep.

6. Increases metabolism – Exercise burns calories, but it also increases your metabolic rate long after you are finished exercising. This helps with energy balance in our bodies and maintaining a healthy weight.

7. Increases energy – I can attest to exercise helping me feel more energetic. If I don't exercise for days in a row, I start to feel the energy drain. Once I get moving again, I feel the energy and motivation return. According to the Mayo Clinic, exercise delivers oxygen and nutrients to your tissues and helps your cardiovascular system work more efficiently. And when your heart and lung health improve, you have more energy to tackle daily chores.

Physical activity goals for adults include at least 150 minutes of moderate intensity aerobic exercise every week. This could be 30 minutes for 5 days or other combinations to equal 150 minutes. Moderate intensity is described as exercise that gets your heart beating faster. Guidelines also include at least 2 days per week of muscle strengthening exercise and stretching exercises to improve flexibility.

If you are not up to this level of an exercise routine, do what you can. Even five minutes of physical activity has real health benefits. So, start where you are, and always check with your health provider for guidance about what is healthy for you. Remember, progress not perfection.

An exercise I teach others is mindful walking. It's walking slowly and paying attention to each step and to your surroundings. Walking this way is good for developing awareness, and it calms and focuses the mind. It's great if you have difficulty with sitting meditations. It's something that can be done any time you walk and helps to bring meditative awareness into daily life and daily activities.

Activate Your Metabolism

Exercise plays a role in metabolism. Energy metabolism includes all the reactions by which the body obtains and spends the energy from food. Basal metabolism is the energy needed to support life when a body is at rest.

Most of the energy burned in a day is for basal metabolism. With aging, the basal metabolic rate slows down. That's why if you eat the same number of calories in your 30s and beyond as you did when you were in your teens or 20s, without increasing your activity level, you will gain weight. This weight gain is often called "creeping overweight."

You may have noticed that people have varying metabolic rates. The person with a high metabolism may seem like they can eat anything and never gain weight, while the person with a slow metabolism seems to gain weight by eating only very little. Genetics is a factor in our metabolism, but there are things we can do to influence it.

Here are some tips to help keep your metabolism functioning at its best:

- Eat breakfast – Eating breakfast enables you to break your nighttime fast, which helps to jump-start your metabolism for the day. Also, breakfast eaters tend to be less hungry all day long and less impulsive about unhealthy snacking.

- Eat regularly – Skipping meals slows metabolism, causing you to burn less calories and store more calories as fat. Also, you tend to eat more later, especially less healthy choices.

- Exercise regularly – Exercise burns calories, but it also helps keep your metabolism higher for hours after you finish your workout. Also, exercise helps to build lean muscle tissue, which burns more calories than fat tissue. With age, your body naturally increases fat and becomes less lean. Exercise helps you maintain or build muscles, so you burn more calories.

<u>Dig Deeper</u>

Reflection and action:

1. Are you eating within the first two hours of waking up to "break your fast?"

2. Are you including exercise in your routine, some or most days of the week? If not, how could you incorporate movement into your daily routine to help keep your metabolism working at its best?

3. Have you ever taken a mindful walk with slow steps and awareness of all around you, noticing what you see and hear along the way? Make awareness of your surroundings the goal instead of how fast or how far you go.

Resources and reading:

1. The United States Department of Health and Human Services Executive Summary Physical Activity Guidelines for Americans (2nd Edition) - https://health.gov/sites/default/files/2019-10/PAG_ExecutiveSummary.pdf

TIP 47 - BE CREATIVE

"Creativity is contagious, pass it on."
Albert Einstein, physicist

"You can't use up creativity. The more
you use, the more you have."
Maya Angelou, poet and writer

You do not have to be an artist to be creative. Growing up, I never saw myself as creative because I was not artistic. My mom and my dad were in health care. Science, not art, seemed to be my destiny. So, there were not many arts and craft projects happening at home. As a result, I shied away from art classes. It wasn't until college that I took a required art class, and, to my surprise, I loved it. For the first time, I felt good doing it. That may have been the first time I realized that it feels good to create art, even if the result doesn't qualify as quality art.

As an adult, I took a class offered through our local arts council called "The Art of Wellness." In the class, we explored various forms of artistic expression and learned about how creating art has been shown, through evidence-based research, to improve various health problems. The class was taught by a local physician, Dr. Mike Weddle, who had completed certification through the Center for Mind-Body Medicine. I had already taken his class "Writing into Wellness" and loved that class. These two classes set me on the course that led me to the Center for Mind-Body Medicine and my own certification. Writing will be addressed in the next tip.

The expressive arts have long been associated with healing. There are fields devoted to using the arts as healing including drama and play therapy, art therapy, music therapy, and dance therapy. In these therapies, self-expression is used as part of treatment, counseling, rehabilitation to achieve healing, growth, and development.

In the eight-week mind-body skills groups that I facilitate using the model from the Center for Mind-Body Medicine, we use three drawings to express: 1) where we are in the moment, 2) our biggest problem, and 3) how we would feel if our biggest problem was resolved.

After a few minutes of deep breathing, insight comes to me every time and I'm able to draw each picture. I have received many inspirations through this process. The deep breathing helps us to pause and search within, and the act of drawing seems to stimulate the brain to go in a direction that helps bring insights not previously identified, from the subconscious to the conscious.

Every week for eight weeks, we practice and learn about mind-body medicine skills and share these with group members. During our last session, we draw three new pictures based on: 1) where we are at the moment, 2) where or who or how you would like to be, and 3) how you will get from where you are to where you want to be. Then we revisit our first three drawings. It's an amazing process that has propelled me toward achieving my goals.

In his book *The Transformation*, Dr. James Gordon shares a powerful and uplifting story of a child he worked with in Gaza after their 2014 war. This story was shared and a young girl who participated in the mind-body skills groups was interviewed by Scott Pelley, for a *60 Minutes* news story about the work of the Center for Mind-Body Medicine in Gaza. The work included children who had lost parents. In the first mind-body skills group, one young girl who was interviewed had initially drawn herself wanting to be killed so she could be with her father, whom she loved but had been killed.

After completing nine, two-hour mind-body skills groups over nine weeks, she learned a variety of the skills I'm discussing in this section, including soft belly breathing, meditation, writing, and drawing. In her drawings on the last day, she no longer saw herself wanting to die, but instead she drew herself as a physician helping to heal people and attending medical school as the way to get there. The words and drawings of the children demonstrated the devastation they had experienced, and the power of the mind-body medicine skills helped heal trauma and restore hope.

The insights gained from these drawings prove that you do not have to be an artist, in the traditional sense of the word, to benefit from using art to express your feelings. You just need to be willing to explore the artistic creativity that is inside you, awaiting an opportunity for expression.

According to the American Art Therapy Association, "art therapy engages the mind, body, and spirit in ways that are distinct from verbal articulations alone." One way to help you understand your own relationship with food is through drawing.

Try incorporating the creative arts into your life to help you better express and understand yourself, and to reach your goals. You will feel better in the process, too!

Dig Deeper
Reflection and action:

1. What creative ways do you express yourself? Do you practice these regularly?

2. Draw your relationship with food. What insights are revealed in your drawing that may help you improve your relationship with food?

Resources and reading:

1. Gordon, J.S. (2019). *The Transformation.* Harper One.

2. Malchiodi, C. (2014). Creative Arts Therapy and Expressive Arts Therapy. *Psychology Today.* https://www.psychologytoday.com/intl/blog/arts-and-health/201406/creative-arts-therapy-and-expressive-arts-therapy

TIP 48 - WRITE OR JOURNAL

"Writing comes as a result of a very strong impulse, and when it does come, I, for one, must get it out."

C.S. Lewis, British writer

I often write to "get it out." In doing so, I am improved in many ways. Most of my life, my writing consisted of school reports, nutrition education handouts, nutrition articles, blog posts, journaling, poetry, and prayers. Many years ago, I realized I felt better after journaling or writing poetry. But I didn't realize writing could help me discover personal insights. I only studied the many medical benefits of writing when I stumbled upon a "Writing into Wellness" class.

I had planned on taking a creative writing class, but it was canceled. At the same time, the college was offering a "Writing into Wellness" class taught by Dr. Mike Weddle. Having worked in wellness for most of my career, this sounded intriguing, so I registered. During the class, we discussed evidence-based research studies showing a connection between expressive writing, health, and improvement in various physical disease symptoms. Some research on the role of writing and health reveals the following health benefits:

- improves lung function in people with asthma
- improves pain and physical health in cancer patients
- improves immune response in people with HIV
- leads to decreased hospitalizations in people with cystic fibrosis
- decreases disease severity in people with rheumatoid arthritis
- improves sleep
- helps with depression and trauma recovery

These are powerful benefits found in writing about your feelings and emotions! As Robert Frost said, "I have never started a poem yet whose end I knew. Writing a poem is discovering."

During one of the most challenging times in my life, I turned to writing poetry. This was something enjoyable to me in child-hood, but for many years I only wrote poems for special oc-casions. When life seemed to be falling apart all around me, I often woke up in the middle of the night to write poem prayers expressing my distress and praying for resolutions. I found great comfort in expressing the cries of my heart. I've included one of these poem prayers at the end of this section.

My clients keep food logs or journals to help provide insights into daily food and beverage intake. Feelings can be added to the food log to help better understand how a food influences your feelings after you eat. How hungry are you when you eat? How full are you when you're finished? Do you feel bloated, tired, or sick after eating? Do you have abdominal pain or changes in bowel habits? Do you feel energized?

Writing down how you feel after a meal and even over the next 24 hours can provide insights that help you feel your best. You are able to identify foods that don't agree with you. Writing about stresses in your day and tying them together with your food choices help identify patterns of behavior you may want to change. Reaching for your pen and paper supplies a healthier way to manage stress than reaching for sweets or other treats.

Dig Deeper

Reflection and action:

1. Keep food logs that include hunger, fullness, and feelings after you eat that day or night, and even the next full day.

2. Keep pen and paper on your nightstand for journaling your feelings.

Resources and reading:

1. Gordon, J.S. (2019). *The Transformation.* Harper One.

2. The Center for Mind-Body Medicine's Dialogue with a Symptom - https://cmbm.org/thetransformation/resources/

3. Salmansohn, K. (2019). *Listen to your Heart: A Line-a-Day Journal.* Andrews McMeel Publishing.

TIP 49 - BE AWE-STRUCK AND
GET OUTSIDE IN NATURE

"You know the feeling when you see a beautiful
sunset or a rainbow. That is the feeling of awe."

Author Unknown

Studies show that the feeling of awe and the experiences that inspire it, help us in many ways, including improving health and relationships. Researchers have found that "awe experiences" increase our prosocial behaviors, making us feel generous and humble. They increase our empathy, making us more willing to trust and connect with others.

An experience of awe involves feeling that you're in the presence of something vast that challenges your understanding of the world. It might be triggered by an encounter with nature, a religious experience, a concert, or sports event. It comes from extraordinarily inspiring experiences in life and in nature, such as the birth of a child, watching a meteor shower, and visiting national parks.

Dacher Keltner, director of the Berkeley Social Interaction Lab, wrote that people report having three awe experiences a week on average. Dr. Keltner's lab has been working with the Sierra Club to take 56 inner-city high-school students on rafting trips and study whether they experience academic benefits. Preliminary findings show that a week after the trip, the teens reported being more engaged and curious.

Awe experiences may help fight depression and reduce inflammation. Researchers believe awe is powerful because it takes us out of our own heads. "Awe minimizes our individual identity and attunes us to things bigger than ourselves," says Paul Piff, assistant professor of psychology at the University of

California.

Author Florence Williams shows how time in nature is not a luxury but is essential for our humanity. During a conference I attended that was led by Florence, we spent the day, which included a walk outdoors, learning about the extensive research on the topic of the health benefits of being in nature. She has traveled around the world studying nature's health benefits, including "forest bathing" in Korea, an "ecotherapeutic" approach to caring for the mentally ill in Scotland, a river trip in Idaho with Iraqi vets suffering from Post-Traumatic Stress Disorder (PTSD), and how being outside helps children with PTSD. It's fascinating research and underscores the importance of getting out in nature and experiencing the awe-inspiring beauty found there.

For me, learning these health benefits convinced me that it is not a matter of going outside when I have time, but it's important to make time to get outside for better health.

Dig Deeper

Reflection and action:

1. When was the last time you were awestruck?

2. Make a list of your favorite things to do in nature and begin incorporating them into your daily or weekly routine.

Resources and reading:

1. Williams, F. (2017). *The Nature Fix: Why Nature Makes Us Healthier, Happier, and More Creative.* W. W. Norton & Company.

2. Emamzadeh, A. (2018). The Psychology of Awe: Awe in Nature. *Psychology Today.* https://www.psychologytoday.com/us/blog/finding-new-home/201807/the-psychology-awe-awe-in-nature

3. Berkeley Social Interaction Lab Website - https://bsil.berkeley.edu/

4. The Greater Good Science Center at University of California, Berkeley - https://greatergood.berkeley.edu/

TIP 50 - IMAGINE AND VISUALIZE

> "Imagination is better than knowledge. For knowledge is limited to all we now know and understand, while imagination embraces the entire world, and all there ever will be to know and understand."
>
> *Albert Einstein, physicist*

> "If you can imagine it, you can achieve it. If you believe it, you can become it."
>
> *William Arthur Ward, writer*

In college, William Arthur Ward's above quote was on a poster in my friend's dorm room with a photo of a ballet dancer leaping beautifully in the air. As a ballet student myself, everything about it inspired confidence, strength, and beauty. Away from home for the first time, I hung on to that quote. It has inspired me ever since.

Imagery has been used by sports psychologists for years. They tell baseball players to imagine the bat striking the ball and seeing it fly over the wall for a home run. Similarly, long distance runners are coached to imagine being the first to cross the finish line. The power of imagining success is an important part of training.

Dr. James Gordon discusses the powerful nature of imagery as the language of our unconscious mind. "People of all ages have used imagery to decrease anxiety and pain, enhance digestive functioning and immunity, promote mental concentration, and alleviate depression. Imagery... reduces the biological and psychological symptoms of post-traumatic stress."

The National Center for Complementary and Integrative Health (part of NIH) is the federal government's lead agency for research on the medical systems, practices, and products that are not considered part of conventional medicine. They define, through rigorous scientific investigation, the usefulness and safety of complementary and integrative health interventions, and their roles in improving health.

Their website defines guided imagery as "a practice used for healing or health maintenance that involves a series of relaxation techniques followed by the visualization of detailed images, usually calm and peaceful in nature."

Have you used imagery to help you in any way? Imagery helps me at doctors' appointments, when giving blood, and getting shots. I hate needles. But every year, I get my flu shot and have lab work done to assess my health, despite my anxiety. For years, I've used imagery to try to transport myself out of the stressful chair I'm sitting in and onto a beautiful, relaxing beach, with waves gently coming in and going out, while I'm resting on warm, soft sand. This is what I do to make the task of the shot or the needle bearable. I noticed after increasing my practice of mind-body medicine skills, including visualization and imagery, I am more quickly transported to that beach and more relaxed for both of these unpleasant activities.

The more you practice, the better you will become at using them as "go-to" help in times of stress. These skills will more readily help you to activate your parasympathetic nervous system, your "rest and digest" antidote to the sympathetic nervous system's "fight or flight" response.

When I'm sitting in the dentist's chair getting my teeth cleaned, I use the same visualization of the beach and add phrases such as, "My legs are heavy and warm, I am at peace," imagining the sun warming me as I relax on the beach. These skills help me to bear the unnerving sound of the dentist's drill and awful scraping of the tools on my teeth.

Another way I've used visualization is to replace unpleasant images with pleasant images. For example, my mind sometimes brings up images of unpleasant and stress-inducing memories. When I see these in my mind's eye, I replace the unpleasant image with one that brings me peace. A counselor once asked me, "What is an image that brings you peace every time you see it?" My first thought was of a familiar picture I saw of Jesus hugging the little children. I saw this picture many times growing up. For many years now, whenever any awful image comes to my mind, I automatically replace it with Jesus hugging the little children and the unpleasant imagery is gone, and so are the unpleasant feelings associated with it.

Visualization and imagery can help improve your eating and health habits. As I mentioned in Tip 38, a stop sign is a powerful visual to help you stop the negative "all or nothing" thinking, such as "I already ate 3 cookies, I might as well eat the whole box." Set your exercise clothes out at night and visualize yourself getting up and going for a walk. Visualize yourself walking past the bakery section in the grocery store without stopping to pick up high sugar desserts. Listen to guided imagery when stressed, instead of going to the kitchen looking for something to eat.

Dig Deeper

Reflection and action:

1. How do you use visualization and imagery in your life?

2. How could you use visualization and imagery more often to help you manage stress and achieve your goals?

Resources and reading:

1. Gordon, J.S. (2019). *The Transformation.* Harper One.

2. The Center for Mind-Body Medicine Website Resources - https://cmbm.org/thetransformation/resources/

3. The National Institutes of Health (NIH) National Center for Complementary and Integrative Health. https://www.nccih.nih.gov/

4. Insight Timer has many guided imagery meditations for sleep, stress, anxiety, and more. www.insighttimer.com.

TIP 51 - BE GRATEFUL

"In everything give thanks."
I Thessalonians 5:18

"Enough is as good as a feast."
Mary Poppins

Gratitude is a strong feeling of appreciation to someone or something for what they have done to help you. I've heard it said that you cannot be angry and grateful at the same time. Gratitude displaces anger. Gratitude brings with it positive mental and physical responses, instead of negative ones, such as those triggered by the fight and flight response. Gratitude changes our brains. Research shows that gratitude unshackles us from toxic emotions and has lasting positive effects on our brains.

Gratitude is Transformative

I started keeping a gratitude journal about 5 years ago. My goal is to write at least 3 things I'm grateful for daily. It serves as a diary or journal that focuses on my blessings. I may not be able to see something positive in my day at first glance, but this motivates me to look for the good, even on the rough and disappointing days. It helps me to look for what Karen Salmansohn calls the "blessons." When you see the blessing in a painful lesson, that's the "blesson." Those are as important as the blessings.

Author Ann Voskamp writes about how a friend of hers challenged her to write one thousand things she was thankful for and how this experience changed her life. She encourages others to live a life of "thanks-living."

I attended a full-day seminar on gratitude with M.J. Ryan,

the author of *Attitudes of Gratitude*. She began the day by asking us to raise our hands if we felt stressed. Almost all 200 participants raised their hands. She then encouraged us to sit back in our seats, close our eyes, and relax. She played the song, "What a Wonderful World" by Louis Armstrong. After the song finished, she asked us to raise our hands if we felt less stressed than we did previously. Almost everyone raised their hands. She pointed out to us that we could change our stress level in just 3 minutes by changing our focus. It was a compelling lesson about the power of gratitude, good thoughts, and music.

Growing up, we said grace before each meal. "Bless us, oh Lord, and these thy gifts, which we are about to receive, from thy bounty, through Christ our Lord, Amen." As an adult, I learned that many families ask a blessing or give thanks, in their own words. Pausing to give thanks, saying grace, or asking a blessing before meals helps to focus our attention on gratitude. We give thanks to God, the farmers, all those who had their hands in bringing our food and preparing it for us. It is a pause that helps us to eat our food more mindfully, with a heart of gratitude.

Dig Deeper

Reflection and action:

1. Keep your own gratitude journal. Buy a blank journal or buy one with inspirational quotes to spark your thoughts.

2. Pause to give thanks, ask a blessing, or say grace before your meals.

Resources and reading:

1. Ryan, M. J. (1999). *Attitudes of Gratitude: How to Give and Receive Joy Every Day of Your Life.* Conari Press.

2. Brown, J., & Wong, J. (2017, June 6). How Gratitude Changes You and Your Brain. *Greater Good Maga-*

zine. https://greatergood.berkeley.edu/article/item/
how_gratitude_changes_you_and_your_brain

3. Voskamp, A. (2011). *One Thousand Gifts: Dare to Live Right Where You Are.* Zondervan.

TIP 52 - PRAY AND KEEP THE FAITH

"Faith is taking the first step, even when you
can't see the whole staircase."

*The Reverend Martin Luther King, Jr., American minister
and civil rights activist*

Since I was a little girl, I've heard prayer referred to as "talking with God." For me, it's a daily running conversation. An article published in the *Indian Journal of Psychiatry* on prayer and healing, stated that "Prayer is a special form of meditation and may therefore convey all the health benefits that have been associated with meditation." These benefits include helping to lower blood pressure, slow aging, and help us think more clearly. They also help to improve concentration, relaxation, digestive problems, reduce symptoms of anxiety, depression, insomnia, stress, and fatigue.

Prayer is certainly a main theme in the Bible and is estimated to be mentioned over 600 times. In the book of Philippians, we are instructed to pray about everything instead of worrying about anything.

I started keeping a prayer journal a couple of years ago. In it, I write my personal prayer requests and the prayer requests of my family and friends. I use this as a guide to help me remember to pray specifically. I leave a space by each request to include the date this prayer was answered or to check it off when no longer a concern. This helps my prayer life to be more relevant and consistent. It helps me to be more faithful in prayer for others and helps me feel better connected with the people in my life. I also add special quotes, scriptures that speak to my heart, and lessons on prayer I read or hear and want to remember.

Two of my favorite prayers are the Lord's Prayer and the

Serenity Prayer, which I include here as a quick prayer for daily living.

The Serenity Prayer

God grant me the serenity to accept the things I cannot change,
The courage to change the things I can,
And the wisdom to know the difference.

Reinhold Niebuhr

I think it is fitting to end with a tip on faith, an anchor, and important part of my life. My faith is in a loving, gracious, and generous God who strengthens and sustains me.

My life has included wonderful blessings, as well as challenges and disappointments. Things haven't always gone the way I wanted them to go. Can you relate? Believing in a loving God and a larger purpose fills my days with hope.

I was raised Catholic and attended Catholic school from kindergarten through 12th grade. Faith has always been an important part of my life. My faith has deepened and become more personal as the years have gone by. I've experienced what it means to believe in someone I cannot see, and who, like the wind, I feel and experience in my daily life.

Did you know that faith and a healthy, long life are connected? When researcher and author Dan Buettner and his team travelled the world researching the places where people live the longest and healthiest lives, one of the nine common denominators, or "principles," they identified among those places was faith.

For their research, they interviewed 263 centenarians, people 100 or more years old. All but five of them belonged to a faith-based community. Dan Buettner writes, "In all Blue Zones regions, centenarians were part of a religious community. People who pay attention to their spiritual side have lower rates of cardiovascular disease, depression, stress, and suicide, and their immune system seems to work better...it allows them to relinquish the stresses of everyday life to a higher power."

I can certainly vouch that this is true in my life. As I was encouraged to do many years ago, I encourage you to seek for yourself. It is healthy to nurture your spiritual side.

Dig Deeper

Reflection and action:

1. Do you pray? Do you have a faith practice?

2. Seek to give prayer and faith a place of importance in your life if you haven't already.

Resources and reading:

1. Lamott, A. (2012). *Help, thanks, wow: The three essential prayers.* Riverhead Books.

2. Shriver, M. (2018). *I've been thinking...reflections, prayers, and meditations for a meaningful life.* Penguin Publishing Group.

3. Moore, B. (2016). *Praying god's word Day by Day.* Broadman and Holman Publishers.

4. Lotz, A. (2020). *The light of his presence.* Multnomah.

5. Andrade C., & Radhakrishnan, R. (2009). Prayer and healing: A medical and scientific perspective on randomized controlled trials. *Indian Journal of Psychiatry*, 51(4):247-53. https://www.doi.org/10.4103/0019-5545.58288

6. Buettner, D. (2012). *The blue zones, second edition: 9 lessons for living longer from the people who've lived the longest.* National Geographic Society.

POEM - GRATEFUL

* * *

Grateful
By Theresa Yosuico Stahl

Grateful for my family
Grateful for my friends
Grateful for the love of God
That never ever ends.

Thankful for the nourishment
Of my daily bread
Mindful that through many hands
I have been well fed.

Overflowing heart
Overflowing mind
Overflowing streams of joy
With beauty of all kinds.

Joyful in the journey
Climbing each new hill
Basking in the sweet sunshine
Laughing, dancing still.

Hopeful for tomorrow
Peaceful in today
Growing, dreaming, loving, learning
All along the way.

CONCLUSION

Over 25 years ago, my desire to write a book was born. Then life happened, as they say. The dream remained, but my life and career took me in different directions. I would return to the book idea on and off over the next two decades. An early retirement offer, and the COVID-19 pandemic prompted me to turn my attention back to book writing.

A lot has happened since that initial idea, both in my personal life and in the nutrition field I entered 40 years ago. My love of food remains. I continue to garden, support local farmers, exercise, get outdoors, and enjoy the natural beauty around me. I raised two adventurous eaters who enjoy local food, gardening, exercise, and the great outdoors. I completed my certification in mind-body medicine. Research continues to shine a spotlight on the importance of nutrition in health, and in the prevention and treatment of disease.

My desire is to pass on some lessons learned. My initial book idea evolved into this simple book of tips, covering the topics that have risen to the top.

1. Food is nourishment and pleasure. Savor it and enjoy every bite.

2. Eat more vegetables and fruits. Make them the stars of the meal and at least half of your plate.

3. Eat mindfully. Eat foods that help you feel your best, move your best, think your best, and look your best. Eat until you are satisfied and full, but not overly full.

4. Food in sight is on your mind. Food out of sight is out of your mind. Make the healthy choice the easy choice.

5. Do unto others as you would have them do unto you. Remember to also do unto yourself as you would do unto others. Be kind to yourself and others.

6. Make time for things you love for stress management. Exercise and move in ways that are enjoyable for you, breathe deeply, meditate, pray, laugh, sleep well, create, and get out in nature. Don't wait until you feel you have time. Make time.

7. Be full: grateful, mindful, joyful, hopeful, faithful, prayerful, thoughtful, and thankful.

Thank you for sharing this journey with me. I'm full.

Please keep in touch at RemindfulEating.com or email me at RemindfulEating@gmail.com.

Also, you can find me on social media:

Facebook: facebook.com/remindfuleating

Instagram: instagram.com/remindfuleating

LinkedIn: linkedin.com/in/theresastahlrdn

RESOURCES AND READING LIST

Part 1

Tip 2
- Wansink, B. (2011). *Mindless eating: Why we eat more than we think.* Hay House.

Tip 3
- David, S. (2016) Emotional agility: Get unstuck, embrace change, and thrive in work and life. Avery.

Tip 4
- Department of Agriculture and U.S. Department of Health and Human Services. *Dietary Guidelines for Americans, 2020-2025.* 9th Edition. December 2020. Available at https://www.dietaryguidelines.gov/resources/2020-2025-dietary-guidelines-online-materials

- Physical Activity Guidelines for Americans - https://health.gov/our-work/nutrition-physical-activity/physical-activity-guidelines/current-guidelines

- Food Marketing Terms - https://www.eatright.org/food/nutrition/nutrition-facts-and-food-labels/understanding-food-marketing-terms

- How much to include on your plate - https://www.myplate.gov/myplate-plan

- Centers for Disease Prevention and Control Newsroom. *Only 1 in 10 adults get enough fruits or vegetables.* https://www.cdc.gov/media/releases/2017/p1116-fruit-vegetable-consumption.html

Tip 5
- Buettner, D. (2012) *The blue zones: second edition: 9 lessons for*

living longer from the people who've lived the longest. National Geographic.

- Salmansohn, K. (2018). *Life is long: 50+ ways to help you live a little bit closer to forever.* 10 Speed Press.

- Salmansohn, K. (2020). *Happy habits: 50 science-backed rituals to adopt (or stop) to boost health and happiness.* 10 Speed Press.

Tip 6
- The Academy of Nutrition and Dietetics. Find a Nutrition Expert in your area - https://www.eatright.org/find-an-expert

- National Eating Disorder Association (NEDA) - https://www.nationaleatingdisorders.org/

- 20 Ways to Love Your Body compiled by Margo Maine on NEDA website – https://tinyurl.com/mpnvwr6d

- Centers for Disease Control and Prevention. *Losing Weight.* https://www.cdc.gov/healthyweight/losing_weight/index.html

Tip 7
- Rolls, B., & Hermann, M. (2012). *The Ultimate Volumetrics Diet: Smart, simple, science-based strategies for losing weight and keeping it off.* William Morrows Cookbooks.

- Seale, S.A., Sherard, T., & Fleming, D. (2010). *The Full Plate Diet.* Bard Press.

Tip 8
- The definition of healthy eating is copyright as follows: ©2016 by Ellyn Satter published at www.EllynSatterInstitute.org.

- Satter, E. (2008). *Secrets of feeding a healthy family: How to eat, how to raise good eaters, 2nd edition.* Kelcy Press.

Tip 9
- For further reading on mindful eating, I recommend books by Dr. Susan Albers and her website - www.eatingmindfully.com.

- Centers for Disease Prevention and Control - https://www.cdc.gov/nchs/products/databriefs/db360.htm

Tip 10
- Tribole, E. & Resch, E. (2012). *Intuitive eating.* St. Martin's Griffin.

- Whitney, E. & Rolfes, S.R. (2013). *Understanding nutrition.* Wadworth, Cengage Learning.

- Wansink, B. (2014). *Slim by design: Mindless eating solutions for everyday life.* William Morrow.

Tip 11
- The Academy of Nutrition and Dietetics. Find a Nutrition Expert in your area - https://www.eatright.org/find-an-expert.

- Wansink, B. (2014). *Slim by design: Mindless eating solutions for everyday life.* William Morrow.

Tip 12
- Krieger, E., & James-Enger, K. (2013). *Small changes, big results. Revised and updated edition.* Clarkson Potter.

Tip 14
- Tribole, E. & Resch, E. (2012). *Intuitive eating.* St. Martin's Griffin.

- Buettner, D. (2012). *The blue zones, second edition: 9 lessons for living longer from the people who've lived the longest.* National Geographic Society.

<u>Tip 15</u>
- Albers, S. (2012). *Eating mindfully, 2nd Edition.* New Harbinger Publications.

- The Slow Food Movement in the USA, visit www.slowfoodusa.org.

<u>Tip 16</u>
- Kristeller, J. (2015). *The Joy of half a cookie.* ORION.

- Albers, S. (2019). *Hanger management: Master your hunger and improve your mood, mind, and relationships.* Little, Brown Spark.

Part 2

<u>Tip 17</u>
- Archibald, A. (2019). *The genomic kitchen.* Amanda Archibald.

- The Academy of Nutrition and Dietetics. Find a Nutrition Expert in your area - https://www.eatright.org/find-an-expert

<u>Tip 18</u>
- Oldways website – www.oldwayspt.org

- Oldways Common Ground Consensus Statement on Healthy Eating – https://oldwayspt.org/programs/oldways-common-ground/oldways-common-ground-consensus

- Winne, M. (2017). *Stand together or starve alone: Unity and chaos in the U.S. food movement.* Praeger.

- Winne, M. (2019). *Food town USA: Seven unlikely cities that are changing the way we eat.* Island Press.

<u>Tip 19</u>
- Beuttner, D. (2017). *Blue zones solution.* National Geographic, 2017.

- Linja, S.S. & Safaii-Waite, S. (2017). *The Alzheimer's prevention food guide.* Rockridge Press.

- Moon, M. (2016). *The mind diet.* Ulysses Press.

- Moon, M. (2019). *The telomere diet and cookbook* by Maggie Moon. Ulysses Press.

- Raffetto, M., & Peterson, W.J. (2017). *Mediterranean diet cookbook for dummies.* For Dummies.

- Patel, G. (2011). *Blending science with spices.* Feeding Health.

- Blatner, D.J. (2010). *The flexitarian diet: The mostly vegetarian way to lose weight, be healthier, prevent disease, and add years to your life.* McGraw-Hill Education.

- Salmansohn, K. (2018). *Life is long.* Ten Speed Press.

Tip 20
- The Human Microbiome Project of the National Institutes of Health (NIH) - https://commonfund.nih.gov/hmp/

Tip 21
- Krieger, E. & James-Enger, K. (2013). *Small changes, big results. Revised and updated.* Clarkson Potter.

Tip 22
- Wansink, B. (2014). *Slim by design: Mindless eating solutions for everyday life.* William Morrow.

- National Institutes of Health's Portion Distortion Quiz - https://www.nhlbi.nih.gov/health/educational/wecan/eat-right/portion-distortion.htm

- Young, L. (2019). *Finally full, finally slim: 30 days to permanent weight loss one portion at a time.* Center Street.

Tip 23
- Rolls, B. & Hermann, M. (2012). *The ultimate volumetrics diet: Smart, simple, science-based strategies for losing weight and keeping it off.* William Morrows Cookbooks.

- Seale, S.A., Sherard, T., & Fleming, D. (2010). *The full plate diet.* Bard Press.

Tip 24
- Krieger, E. & James-Enger, K. (2013). *Small changes, big results. Revised and updated.* Clarkson Potter.

Tip 25
- Tribole, E. & Resch, E. (2012). *Intuitive eating.* St. Martin's Griffin.

- Wansink, B. (2011). *Mindless eating: Why we eat more than we think.* Hay House.

Tip 26
- Krieger, E. (2009). *So easy.* John Wiley and Sons.

- Krieger, E. (2019). *Whole in one.* Da Capo Lifelong Books.

- Geagan, K. (2009). *Go green get lean.* Rodale.

- Rust, R. (2022). *Zero waste cooking for dummies.* For Dummies.

Tip 27
- Andrews, L. C. (2021). *Heart healthy meal prep: 6 weekly plans for low-sodium, high-flavor, grab-and-go meals.* Rockridge Press.

- Nicholson, S. (2010). *7-Day menu planner for dummies.* For Dummies.

- USDA MyPlate Recipes with videos and more -
www.myplate.gov/myplate-kitchen/recipes

Tip 29

- Patel, G. (2011). *Blending science with spices.* Feeding Health.

- Amidor, T. (2017). *The healthy meal prep cookbook.* Rockridge Press.

- The James Beard Foundation. (2018). Waste *not: How to get the most from your food.* Rizzoli.

- Excellent resource with practical tools to help families decrease food waste from the United States Environmental Protection Agency. https://www.epa.gov/sustainable-management-food/food-too-good-waste-implementation-guide-and-toolkit#docs

Tip 30

- For farmers' markets close to your home visit www.localharvest.org. To find a farmers' market in your area visit: https://www.ams.usda.gov/local-food-directories/farmersmarkets.

- Your Guide to Physical Activity and Your Heart. U.S. Department of Health and Human Services, National Institutes of Health, National Heart, Lung, and Blood Institute 2006 https://www.nhlbi.nih.gov/files/docs/public/heart/phy_active.pdf

- Haugen, J. (2016). *The mom's guide to a nourishing garden.* https://jenhaugen.com/book/

- NPR - https://www.npr.org/sections/thesalt/2012/02/17/147050691/can-gardening-help-troubled-minds-heal.

- Forrest K., & Stuhldreher W. (2011). Prevalence and correlates of vitamin D deficiency in US adults. *Nutrition Research, 31*(1), 48-54. https://www.doi.org/10.1016/j.nutres.2010.12.001

Tip 31
- Produce for Better Health "Have a Plant" campaign - https://fruitsandveggies.org/

- Palmer, S. (2012). *The plant powered diet.* The Experiment.

Tip 32
- Harvard Health Publishing. (2019, November 5). *The sweet danger of sugar.* https://www.health.harvard.edu/heart-health/the-sweet-danger-of-sugar

- Quick tips for reading food labels from the Food and Drug Administration: https://www.fda.gov/media/131162/download

Tip 33
- Dietary Reference Intakes - https://ods.od.nih.gov/HealthInformation/Dietary_Reference_Intakes.aspx

- Clark, N. (2019). *Nancy Clark's sports nutrition guidebook.* Human Kinetics.

Tip 34
- Thalheimer, J.C. (2018). The power of coffee. *Today's Dietitian*, 20(3) 20. https://www.todaysdietitian.com/newarchives/0318p20.shtml

Tip 35
- Seale, S.A., Sherard, T., & Fleming, D. (2010). *The full plate diet.* Bard Press.
- Rolls, B., & Hermann, M. (2012). *The ultimate volumetrics diet: Smart, simple, science-based strategies for losing weight and keeping it off.* William Morrows Cookbooks.
- Dietary fiber in common foods - https://www.dietaryguidelines.gov/resources/2020-2025-dietary-guidelines-online-materials/food-sources-select-nutrients/food-0

Tip 36
- Wansink, B. (2014). *Slim by design: Mindless eating solutions for everyday life.* William Morrow.

Tip 37
- The Partnership for Food Safety Education – https://www.fightbac.org/

- The FoodKeeper App and Website - https://www.foodsafety.gov/keep-food-safe/foodkeeper-app

Part 3

Tip 38
- Karen Salmansohn's website and books - www.notsalmon.com

- Newberry, T. (2007). *The 4:8 Principle: The Secret to a Joy-Filled Life.* Tyndale.

Tip 39
- The Moderation Movement – www.moderationmovement.com.au

- The U.S. Weight Loss and Diet Control Market at the Research and Markets online store - https://www.researchandmarkets.com/research/qm2gts/the_72_billion?w=4

- Olshansky, S. Passaro, D., Hershow, R., Layden, J., Carnes, B., Brody, J., Hayflick, L., Butler, R., Allison, D., & Ludwig, D. (2005). A potential decline in life expectancy in the United States in the 21st century. *The New England Journal of Medicine.* Massachusetts Medical Society. https://doi.org/10.1056/NEJMsr043743

Tip 40
- Nerurkar, A., Bitton, A., Davis, R. B., Phillips, R. S., & Yeh, G.

(2013). When physicians counsel about stress: results of a national study. *JAMA Internal Medicine, 173*(1), 76–77. https://doi.org/10.1001/2013.jamainternmed.480

- Fogt, E., & Shah, N. (2014). *Having your all: How self-care leads to an energized, empowered and effective life.* Women Wellness.

Tip 41
- Gordon, J.S. (2019). *The Transformation.* Harper One.

Tip 42
- Russo, M. A., Santarelli, D. M., & O'Rourke, D. (2017). The physiological effects of slow breathing in the healthy human. *Breathe* 13: 298-309.

- Gordon, J.S. (2019). *The Transformation.* Harper One.

Tip 43
- Gordon, J.S. (2019). *The Transformation.* Harper One.

- The Center for Mind-Body Medicine – www.cmbm.org - free meditations to practice under the heading "education" under the "self-care resources" and free webinars under the "webinars" heading in that same section.

- Insight Timer App – www.insighttimer.com

- Calm App – www.calm.com

- Abide Bible and Meditation App – https://abide.co/

- Nerurkar, A., Bitton, A., Davis, R. B., Phillips, R. S., & Yeh, G. (2013). When physicians counsel about stress: results of a national study. *JAMA Internal Medicine, 173*(1), 76–77. https://doi.org/10.1001/2013.jamainternmed.480

Tip 44
- *Mayo Clinic.* Stress Relief from Laughter? It's No Joke. https://

www.mayoclinic.org/healthy-lifestyle/stress-management/in-depth/stress-relief/art-20044456

Tip 45
- American Academy of Sleep Medicine – www.aasm.org

- Sleep Education – www.sleepeducation.org

Tip 46
- The United States Department of Health and Human Services Executive Summary Physical Activity Guidelines for Americans (second edition) - https://health.gov/sites/default/files/2019-10/PAG_ExecutiveSummary.pdf

Tip 47
- Gordon, J.S. (2019). *The Transformation.* Harper One.

- Malchiodi, C. (2014). Creative Arts Therapy and Expressive Arts Therapy. *Psychology Today.* https://www.psychologytoday.com/intl/blog/arts-and-health/201406/creative-arts-therapy-and-expressive-arts-therapy

Tip 48
- Gordon, J.S. (2019). *The Transformation.* Harper One.

- The Center for Mind-Body Medicine's Dialogue with a Symptom - https://cmbm.org/thetransformation/resources/

- Salmansohn, K. (2019). *Listen to your Heart: A Line-a-Day Journal.* Andrews McMeel Publishing.

Tip 49
- Williams, F. (2017). *The Nature Fix: Why Nature Makes Us Healthier, Happier, and More Creative.* W. W. Norton & Company.

- Emamzadeh, A. (2018). The Psychology of Awe: Awe in Nature. *Psychology Today.* https://www.psychologytoday.com/us/

blog/finding-new-home/201807/the-psychology-awe-awe-in-nature

- Berkeley Social Interaction Lab Website - https://bsil.berkeley.edu/

- The Greater Good Science Center at University of California, Berkeley - https://greatergood.berkeley.edu/

Tip 50
- Gordon, J.S. (2019). *The Transformation.* Harper One.

- The Center for Mind-Body Medicine Website Resources - https://cmbm.org/thetransformation/resources/

- The National Institutes of Health (NIH) National Center for Complementary and Integrative Health. https://www.nccih.nih.gov/

- Insight Timer has many guided imagery meditations for sleep, stress, anxiety, and more. www.insighttimer.com

Tip 51
- Ryan, M. J., (1999). *Attitudes of Gratitude: How to Give and Receive Joy Every Day of Your Life.* Conari Press.

- Brown, J., & Wong, J. (2017, June 6). How Gratitude Changes You and Your Brain. *Greater Good Magazine.* https://greatergood.berkeley.edu/article/item/how_gratitude_changes_you_and_your_brain

- Voskamp, A. (2011). *One Thousand Gifts: Dare to Live Right Where You Are.* Zondervan.

Tip 52
- Lamott, A. (2012). *Help, thanks, wow: The three essential prayers.* Riverhead Books.

- Shriver, M. (2018). *I've been thinking...reflections, prayers, and meditations for a meaningful life.* Penguin Publishing Group.

- Moore, B. (2016). *Praying god's word Day by Day.* Broadman and Holman Publishers.

- Lotz., A. (2020). *The light of his presence.* Multnomah.

- Andrade C., & Radhakrishnan, R. (2009). Prayer and healing: A medical and scientific perspective on randomized controlled trials. *Indian Journal of Psychiatry*, 51(4):247-53. https://www.doi.org/10.4103/0019-5545.58288

- Buettner, D. (2012). *The blue zones, second edition: 9 lessons for living longer from the people who've lived the longest.* National Geographic Society.

Note: Nutrition information is based on USDA FoodData Central: https://fdc.nal.usda.gov/fdc-app.html#/

ACKNOWLEDGEMENTS

What a journey! And so many helpers along the way to thank.

Thank you to my clients and class participants who continuously inspire me, laugh with me, and have fed this dream to write a book. Thank you to the RDNs I've worked with who have done the same.

Thank you to my colleagues who have written so many informative, excellent books that I've enjoyed reading over the years. I have highlighted many of your excellent books in my resources and reading section.

Thank you to the writers, teachers, and mentors I've had along the way - those with whom I've had the privilege of learning from in classes, and those I've only known through the pages of your books.

Thank you, Carey Moffatt, for your expert coaching, which helped me to stay motivated and move forward, no matter the pace, and for reminding me that progress is progress. Thank you, Debbie D'Aquino, for your coaching inspiration and steady encouragement.

Thank you to graphic designer, Julie Matheney, for your expert cover designs and Remindful Eating logo, which captured the concepts of my mission (Remind, Mind, Full, Mindful, and Mindful Eating) in one graphic.

Special thanks to my dear dietitian friend and colleague, Cindy

Held. I'm not sure that I would have finished this book without your encouragement and support. You kept the dream alive. You read and reread, and you always provided excellent feedback and editing. I am so grateful.

Thank you to those who also had a hand in editing and proofreading, including Mary Molloy, Julie Beyer, and Katie Hershey. Your input and encouragement meant so much and kept me going. Special thanks to Mark Winne for your expert copyediting and mentoring. You stepped in and saved the day at a critical point in the book's journey.

Thank you to Liz Jalkiewicz, The Dietitian Editor, for stepping into unchartered waters and helping to bring the project home by formatting, proofreading, and assisting in the final stages.

Thank you to my family who inspired my love of food. We spent countless, enjoyable hours around the table filled with flavorful food and love. I cherish those memories. Special thanks to my husband, Jim, and to my children, Sarah and Benjamin. We've shared countless hours in the garden, in the kitchen, around the table, and in conversation about this book - SURPRISE! It's been a long time coming, but each step has had meaning and significance.

Thank you to each reader for choosing this book. I hope it will inspire you to enjoy the pleasures of living a well-nourished life.

ABOUT THE AUTHOR

Theresa Yosuico Stahl

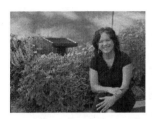 Theresa Yosuico Stahl, RDN, LDN, FAND is passionate about helping people live full and satisfying lives. She has been promoting food as medicine for four decades. Recognizing the powerful relationship between mental and physical health, she completed certification and serves as a supervisor with the Center for Mind-Body Medicine. Theresa is a Fellow of the Academy of Nutrition and Dietetics.

As a registered and licensed dietitian nutritionist and consultant, she provides high-risk nutrition counseling with the Allegany County, Maryland WIC program, and teaches nutrition and facilitates mind-body skills groups with Allegany College of Maryland's Center for Continuing Education. She enjoys connecting with people and speaks and writes on a variety of nutrition and wellness topics locally and nationally.

Theresa served on the nutrition faculty of Potomac State College of West Virginia University. Providing medical nutrition therapy in pediatrician and primary care providers' offices for over half of her career, she values collaboration in health care.

Theresa serves as vice-chair of the Western Maryland Food Council, she is a member of the Maryland Food System Resiliency Council and the University of Maryland Extension Advisory Committee.

Theresa is available for nutrition and wellness presentations. For more information, visit her website https://www.remindfuleating.com, sign up to receive tips, reminders, and recipes, and connect on social media.

Made in the USA
Middletown, DE
27 February 2023

25400899R00128